Hope through the Eyes of Love

Hope through the Eyes of Love

Life and Marriage in the Face of a Brain Tumor

Patricia Meserve Gauvin

and

Angel Logan

To order additional copies of this book, contact:
Xlibris Corporation
1-888-795-4274
www.Xlibris.com
Orders@Xlibris.com
91208

**Credits and heartfelt thanks to
both of these wonderful, talented women.**

Front cover painting
Paradise Found, by **Judy Shillinburg**
http://www.judyshillingburgwatercolors.com

Back cover Author Photo
Jennifer Hansen
http://www.destinphotographer.org/

CONTENTS

Preface

When we say our wedding vows to each other, promising to love the other for better or for worse, for richer or for poorer, in sickness and in health, for as long as we both shall live, we often say these traditional words because that is what people have been saying for generations. We stand before the people who are closest to us and make promises we intend to keep. However, we do not always fully understand the impact of those promises, which is evident by the number of divorces today. Many marry with the option to divorce over insignificant issues, misunderstandings, lack of communication, or other trivial matters. Many marry without truly knowing their partners and build the foundation of their connection upon infatuation rather than love. Of course, there are those who say the words, but when faced with the serious issues of life, they allow fear and uncertainty to drive them apart.

The ideal of marriage sits upon an unstable pedestal because of the ever-changing issues that continually arise within society today. However, its true essence remains unchanged, if we say our vows with the intention of marrying for life and approach every aspect of our marriage with unconditional love and unyielding commitment. If we can accept our partners completely without judgment and deal with the issues and occasional adversity that will inevitably arise, we will have a chance for marital success.

Of course, adversity is like a chameleon, taking on limitless shapes and sizes, while affecting our lives from minor to severe ways. It does not discriminate or target anyone in particular. Adversity simply appears like a hurricane, waiting to cause devastation; and while it is harmful enough, it is our preparation and the resolve, which will determine the outcome. We can easily succumb to the effects of the trials and tribulations of life, but we have a choice to either let it swallow us or to fight back. It sounds simple, but I can assure it is not. However, it is a choice, and we must truly think about what our vows to each other mean and the reasons to make them. Only then can we truly appreciate the sanctity of marriage.

When adversity struck the life I share with my husband, as much as we wanted to wish it away, we had to face the reality of it; and we chose to rise above it, fight for us, and prevail against all odds. Again, it is simple in concept, and it has been anything but simple. However, love and hope can be the glue that holds anyone together, giving you the motivation to triumph.

This is a true story about our remarkable journey in the face of the worst kind of adversity, sharing how we allowed our love for each other to bond us, rather than tear us apart. We have traveled through the forest of fear, loss, and acceptance; but most of all, we found hope in the best place possible—within the eyes of each other.

Dearly Beloved

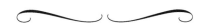

"It is a tumor in the middle of the temporal lobe of his brain about the size of a walnut." That was Dr. Pinto-Lord's response when I asked about the spot that did not belong on my husband, Ron's MRI films. Fear does not even begin to explain the surge of emotions I felt at that moment. It is incomprehensible how one sentence—a collection of words thrown together—could alter someone's entire life in a matter of seconds. One minute, we were invincible together; and the next, we were vulnerable to life's uncertainties.

My husband had just received an earth-shattering diagnosis that should have rendered an emotional outburst, especially at the thought of having a brain tumor. However, he sat calmly, believing with every fiber of his being that he could conquer anything that challenged him—including a brain tumor. This quiet attitude was so characteristic of Ron. Instead of feeling enraged or showing fear and sadness as most people would, he handled the news with strength and courage, willing to meet whatever challenge came his way. I will never forget that day—a fleeting moment when time stood still, long enough to change the course of our lives forever. Ron's reaction to the events of that day was a true testament to his character.

My beloved husband, Ronald Gauvin, was born on June 1, 1958, in Dover, New Hampshire, to Ray and Claire Gauvin. Ron's parents were regular people living regular lives. Fancy was not in their vocabulary, and being practical was a normal way of life. Neither had graduated from high school, and they married young, as many couples did during that era. If you were not wealthy, you did not have a career—you had a job.

The Gauvins were hardworking and honest individuals who were trying to do their best for the family. Claire was happy to stay at home to raise their children, while Ray served his country in the US Navy during World War II. This lifestyle was typical for families at wartime—most wives stayed at home while their husbands served in the military. The husbands rarely had leave, and the kids barely recognized their fathers when they did come home for visits. Fortunately, Ray Gauvin's time in the service was over while the kids were still young. When he returned, he began working as a welder in the local navy yard. This was a grueling job, which kept Ray away from home for many hours each day, but his first priority was to provide for his family. Claire never complained about their circumstances. She simply did her part—to maintain their household. The Gauvins were certainly not wealthy, but dinner was always on the table, and their children always had the essentials.

As with any family during those days, kids came along rather quickly. Ray and Claire Gauvin had two sons and two daughters. Their oldest child was Dickie, followed by Joanne, Ron, and Dianne.

Sadly, in 1961, Ron's twelve-year-old brother, Dickie, died from an accidental gunshot wound when Ron was three and his sister Joanne was ten. This tragedy shook his family to the core and changed the way they viewed life to some degree. Ron learned about loss before any child should. Ron looked up to his older brother and missed him terribly after he died. No one else in the family appeared to be having any outward reactions to Dickie's death, but Ron had a tendency to show his emotions more than anyone else did. Being such a young age, Ron had a difficult time understanding what happened, and he cried whenever he saw pictures of his brother. I think this surprised his parents a little, because many people think that children at that young age are not aware of as much or won't remember everything that happens. However, knowing what I do now about Ron, I think that Dickie's death impacted him much more than anyone realized at the time. I also believe that Ron quietly carried that loss with him throughout life, and it may have affected some of his decisions later.

Ron's parents were devastated because of the loss of their son and the circumstances surrounding the shooting. However, they did not say too much about Dickie's death to the kids or anyone else. Clearly, they were hurting, but they seemed to internalize their pain and showed it in other ways. A child dying during those days was not typical, and when it happened, it caused parents to pause and reevaluate the way they handled the safety of their children. The Gauvins couldn't help but be afraid all of the time, worrying that something could happen to the other kids. Consequently, they became overprotective with their other children because they were afraid that Ron and Joanne might get hurt the way their older brother did. No one talked about the nature of the accident, but it was not too difficult to figure out. Needless to say, Ray and Claire did not permit either child to do any chores or to participate in any activities that could risk their well-being. They were quite adamant about the safety of their children. One would think that a mother might be more cautious, but Ron's father seemed to be more fearful. He was particularly concerned about Ron being hurt around his power tools, the car, or anything that could cause an accident. He never allowed Ron to help with household projects or repairs. Kids in other families had to do chores in and out of the house, but because of this tragedy, the Gauvin kids lived a life of leisure.

Ron's Mom worked part time for most of his childhood to supplement Ray's income and to help support the family. However, a time came when her schedule changed from part-time to full-time hours, which meant she would be away from the home more often. The children were too young to be home alone, so she had to find an appropriate babysitter to care for her kids while she was away. Ron had a tough time adjusting to his mother's extended work hours because he knew it meant less time with her. He may have been a little clingy because he lost his brother and didn't fully understand death. All he knew was that Dickie left and never came back home. Ronnie, as she called him, truly loved his mother, and he really struggled when she had to go to work. He missed her terribly, and when he saw his mother ironing her clothes for work, he cried. Ron and his mother had a particularly close relationship when he was little. She spent as much time with Ron as possible between her domestic duties and her time with Joanne. She was very warm and loving, and played a variety of board and card games with Ron. Of course, she sympathized with her son, but her additional income was necessary to keep up with the household expenses. Considering her dilemma with Ron, she tried to be more selective when searching for a babysitter. She wanted Ron to feel the least amount of anxiety possible in this situation. Amazingly, in a short time, she found an ideal babysitter who was willing to do more than just be an authoritative presence. The babysitter loved the idea of playing games with the kids and giving them the attention they might miss with their mother at work. She made a true effort and this made things much easier for Ron.

Life changed a bit when Ron's little sister, Dianne, came along. Ron welcomed Dianne's arrival and he immediately took his new little sister under his wing. He wanted to protect her from all of the dark elements of the world while loving the role of a big brother. Ron loved his sister, Joanne, and got along great with her, but she was a little older with more interest in doing her own things with friends her own age.

A few years prior, Ron's father had been doing some renovating in the upstairs area of their house to build extra rooms and expand their home for the children, but when Dickie died, Ray Gauvin suddenly stopped his work and boarded up the entire area. I suspect that he intended the first room to be for his son, Dickie. Then, two years later, after Dianne was born, Ron's father decided to open up the upstairs again and continue building the room. When he was finished, the stairs led directly into Ron's room first, and then, there was a door inside of Ron's room that led to Dianne's room, similar to a hotel suite. Ron and Dianne shared a mutual closet that separated the two rooms.

Dianne adored Ron, and she wanted to be everywhere that he went. She could not sleep unless her big brother was upstairs in his room too. The two spent countless hours playing together in their rooms, and if they were not upstairs, they were in the basement playing. Dianne loved it when Ron pretended to be her horse and ran around on his hands and knees with Dianne on his back, clutching a tie around his neck or his belt to keep her from falling off. She giggled endlessly and begged Ron to keep playing.

The Gauvins took several family trips during the weekends or on annual vacation in the summer. They often drove up north to go to the lake or to the mountains. In addition, they loved visiting with relatives when they could. The kids had a great time seeing their extended family, and they enjoyed spending time and playing games with their cousins. When they visited the lake, they had a camp area where they stayed and where they housed their boat. The family had hours of fun in the water, while Ron and Joanne water-skied together, which was right up Ron's alley. Joanne usually needed some help getting up onto her skis, but Ron knew how to do it all himself. He had a blast doing anything in the water, including fishing with his father during the lake trip. Ron appreciated the chance to do something fun with his dad. The Gauvins also traveled to a few other places in New Hampshire, Vermont, and Maine, such as Santa's Village and Storyland. However, a family favorite was Six Gun City, which was an old west theme park up in the White Mountains of New Hampshire. Ron loved visiting Six Gun City with all of the horse drawn carriages, ponies, and the entire western motif. During one trip, Ron found a cowboy whip to play with, and he was having a blast swinging and whipping it around. It was a lot of fun until he accidentally hit Dianne in the eye with it. Ray Gauvin was not having it. He was just as protective with Dianne, as he was with the other two children, and he immediately became unglued. He took the whip away from Ron and never returned it. I think he had let up on the kids a bit until that happened, and he remembered why they had been so protective before.

Ron did not sit still very long. He was bursting with energy and always interested in trying every activity under the sky. He was even in the Boy Scouts, and he did quite well. Ron's mother remembered him as a very well-behaved kid. Other than the minor things that boys did to get under their parents' skin, he did not get into any trouble. Oddly, he was an incredibly neat boy who kept his room clean. She never remembered having to chase him down to clean his room, and he was even tidier than his sisters were. The only problem Ron really had was getting through school, as he struggled during his early years. In fact, the school kept him back in third grade, and he had to see a tutor during the summer to help get him back on track. Math was his worst subject at the time, and as much as he tried, he still had to work twice as hard to get through it. Of course, he met that challenge as he did any others, and rose above it.

Despite the initial struggles with his studies, Ron had many friends while he attended Garrison School. He was friendly, talkative, and loved doing all the things that the boys his age enjoyed doing, such as riding his bike or building forts with his friends. They seemed to enjoy his company just as much.

Unlike other kids, Ron did not seem affected by peer pressure at all. He was a little leader and not a follower. He thought for himself and was never interested in trying to fit into anyone else's groups or cliques. When it came to his little sister, Dianne, he did not hesitate to watch out for her, especially when she started first grade. He felt responsible for her and always kept an eye on Dianne to make sure she was okay at all times.

One day, Dianne dropped her lunch all over the floor in front of everyone and was clearly upset. Ron immediately rushed to her side to help her clean it up. He was in fifth grade at the time, and this was not typical of boys of his age. Most might have let their little sisters deal with it on their own, but not Ron—he loved Dianne and would have done anything for her. Ron did not concern himself with what other kids thought, and I think they were smart enough to know how much he adored his sister, and they probably watched out for her too. After Ron finished helping her clean the food from the floor, he gladly escorted his little sister up to the counter, while holding her hand, to get her a new lunch.

Every day, Ron walked Dianne to the bus stop to make sure she was okay and not alone. He waited until the bus picked her up and then he was on his way. If he and his friends went to the river to go ice-skating, he did not mind taking Dianne along with him. He always helped her put on the skates and helped her along the ice to be sure she was steady. The ironic thing is that Ron's parents were beyond overprotective about every little tiny thing, but they allowed the kids to go ice-skating. To me, that was miraculous considering how protective they were, and how afraid they were of something terrible happening. I couldn't think of anything more terrible than if the kids had fallen through the ice. Of course, I am sure that if his parents had really thought about it, they would not have given their approval and would have put an end to it.

Claire Gauvin's face always lit up when she recalled her son's childhood, and the many pleasant memories of *Ronnie* outside with his friends playing hockey or peewee football. She really enjoyed watching him grow up and interact with his friends. Claire also said that Ron was very artistic. He loved to draw cartoon characters, which is the reason why she let him paint life-sized characters on the wall in his bedroom. He did a great job, and it made his room more suited for a boy at his age. She laughed as she told me about the time he painted an Indian squaw in a canoe. She said it was a beautiful painting, but he drew a naked squaw.

Ron's drawing skills came in handy at holiday time because he loved to make decorations for Christmas, to make the house more festive. There was a regular contest posted in the TV guide back then for people who could draw. Ron drew and submitted pictures for that contest a few times, and he was so excited when they finally responded to him, telling Ron that he had a lot of talent. Many thought that Ron would take his artistic ability into adulthood, but for some reason, he eventually stopped drawing. No one knew the reason why, but he moved on to other interests. Ron continued fishing with his dad because he really enjoyed their quality time together. As much as Ron enjoyed spending time with the women in his family, especially Dianne, he also wanted to have time with his dad to do a men's sport, without any women around them.

Ron's family was not the type to wear their emotions on their sleeves or gush about the love they felt for each other. Yet they seemed to have a silent understanding between them because they clearly loved one another. Ron's father had a more stoic demeanor and showed his love to his family in different ways. For instance, even though Claire Gauvin cooked plenty for everyone to eat at dinnertime, Ray refused to eat a second helping of food until he was sure that everyone else at the table had enough to eat. The kids could have had two and three helpings, but that did not matter to him. He wanted to be sure that they had what they wanted before he took another bite. When other husbands took their wives out for an occasional dinner at a restaurant, Ray never took Claire out to dinner without their children. He wasn't trying to slight his wife at all—he just didn't want to slight his children by enjoying a great dinner out without them. Ray Gauvin had his quirks, and he was a little reminiscent of the television character, Archie Bunker, but not in a negative way—more in humor than anything else. It was his way of loving and connecting with his family without saying the actual words. Evidently, he didn't start saying, "I love you" to the kids until they grew up.

Because Ray was so protective, not wanting Ron to do anything strenuous that could cause him harm, Ron needed to find more to do with his time, so he started pursuing a variety of sports and hobbies. Ron had a strong appreciation for everything that nature had to offer, so he never missed the opportunity to participate in anything outdoor-related. He tried canoeing, biking, fishing, and bow hunting. Ron was exceptionally good at photography. He had a keen eye for outdoor life and loved to capture as much as he could on film. When Ron mastered one hobby, he tried the next, and then the next, and discovered that there were a million things in life that he enjoyed doing.

In high school, Ron was popular among his friends. Everyone knew him, even the kids that were not in his class. The teachers also thought highly of Ron and enjoyed having him in their classes. Ron did much better in his studies when he was in high school. Whenever his younger sister told others that Ron was her brother, they immediately sang his praises and welcomed her warmly because they liked him so much. The funny thing was that Ron and I actually attended the same high school together, but I didn't know Ron personally. I had heard of him and I vaguely remember seeing him around along with other members of his family, but we didn't really travel in the same circle of friends, so we never had the opportunity to meet.

Ron got involved in several sports like track and football. Then, when the high school started their first soccer team, he joined and quickly excelled in soccer. Ron was beyond skilled and he never did anything halfway. He was always willing to meet any challenge with boundless commitment, and he was determined to be the best at everything he tried.

After Ron graduated from high school, he discovered the world of archery—he was definitely in his element. Quite honestly, I don't think he was ever a beginner in archery because within a short period of time, he was winning medal beyond medal in several national archery tournaments.

Ron worked full time at a factory but during his time off, he spent every moment practicing in order to become a skilled archery marksman. Later, he discovered the underwater world and scuba diving. As much as he loved archery, scuba diving had a different effect on him. He loved all of his other hobbies but scuba diving was not just another hobby. Ron realized that it was his passion, and he decided that he wanted to make it his career. Ron finally figured out what he wanted to do with his life. He always had a strong interest in the mysterious world underwater, especially old shipwrecks. He thought it would be cool to uncover the various artifacts and possible treasures, and to learn the history of the ships. Ron envisioned himself combining his skills in photography with scuba diving to create the ultimate career. He was sure that he could capture history frame by frame through every aspect of a shipwreck recovery.

In Florida and the Bahamas, during the mid-eighties, there were many reports in the media about several billion-dollar treasure recovery projects for a variety of historic shipwrecks, and Ron wanted to be part of that excitement. Of course, he knew that the only way he could be successful in this field was to learn everything he could about his prospective career, he wanted to enhance his skills with deep-water gear. Ron thought the best way to achieve his goals was by becoming familiar with all of the people who frequented the local dive shops. He knew that he would learn the most from these individuals, and he absorbed as much as he could. Before long, Ron's ambition and persistence paid off because he and one of his friends found a man with a mutual interest in locating treasure ships. This was music to his ears. Ron and his friend spent several hours planning and dreaming until their big opportunity arrived. The problem was that Ron needed to move to Florida to pursue his dream, which was not necessarily a problem for him, but his parents were a different story. They did not approve of this idea at all. They thought that leaving a good paying job in New Hampshire to chase a dream was being frivolous, and they thought that this idea was more of a fantasy than a real future. Ron's parents could not understand because he had worked at Janco, a factory, for eight years, and then had moved up and became a circuit board welder for Hewlett-Packard. He had some interest in computers, and the skills he had developed would make the Hewlett Packard job the perfect position for him.

His parents weren't trying to take away Ron's dreams; they just wanted him to have a secure future, and they viewed his job with Hewlett Packard as a more reliable path to reach that future. However, despite his parents concern and advice, he was not willing to let go of his scuba diving dream. Ron was willing to move mountains to bring that dream to a reality. When his parents saw Ron's determination, they asked him to put the move on hold until he researched everything and had all of the details worked out. This made sense to Ron because he needed the time to work out the logistics and figure out his finances. Of course, this also gave his parents the time they needed to talk him out of it.

To Love and to Cherish

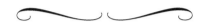

I was born, Patricia Meserve, on July 28, 1960, to Robert and Arlene Meserve of Dover, New Hampshire. My parents shared common backgrounds—both were Irish and French, though my mother was Catholic and my father was Protestant. They were children during the depression and were part of the working-class poor.

I was the sixth of a huge family of nine children, with four brothers and four sisters. My mother's first child was stillborn, and before she gave birth to me, she had a miscarriage with another child, which would have made an even larger family of eleven children.

When I was young, mothers taught their daughters how to do housework and ladylike things. My mother taught me how to clean, cook, sew, fold clothing, and even play piano and trumpet. However, I was not the typical girl at all. I came crashing into the world as an eleven-pound baby, and as I grew up towering over the other girls my age, my interests revolved less around girly things and more around activities like mowing the lawn. Despite my unique differences, my mother allowed me to be myself. When I was too big to sit on her lap, she welcomed my hugs and kisses every night, and she never made me feel odd for being different. Instead, she always made me feel special.

I guess you could say that I was a tomboy because I loved sports. I played kickball with my friends, I went roller-skating, I swam like a fish, and yes, I played football. Sure, I still loved dolls and pretty things, but I could not sit still for very long. I was an active girl, full of drive and curiosity. I remember the astronauts landing on the moon when I was nine, and I was in complete awe. I wondered how they were able to propel a rocket up that high, how they knew how much fuel it would take, and what it was like on the moon. I remembered thinking that if men could go up to the moon and then televise it to all of us here on earth—anything in the world was possible.

I did not give my parents any problems because I liked being the "good girl" and hanging out with the kids who thought the way I did. I wasn't trying to impress anyone; I just didn't see the point of making life hard for myself. Not to mention, I was not shy at all. That may have been because I grew up with so many siblings. You could not be shy if you had something to say in our household.

I loved having so many siblings because I genuinely had fun with my brothers and sisters so much that I didn't feel the need to look for new friends very often. Despite the number of people who lived in our house, I never viewed our family as being very large, and I really appreciated that I could be myself around everyone. Perhaps that is why I had such a strong sense of family, because everything we did was family oriented. I loved the big gatherings at holiday time and I looked forward to seeing all of our extended relatives—I wanted those days to last forever. I think, overall, I had a happy childhood.

I do remember a difficult time when I stayed with my Aunt Blanche who was dying of cancer. She was my great aunt and I was only ten. I guess it was a little unusual for a child my age to be in that position, but I felt comfortable being with her even though the circumstances were very sad. She told me that she had observed me, and she thought I would make a wonderful nurse. This meant so much coming from her because she was a nurse, and she evidently believed that I was caring enough to follow within her footsteps.

She gave me an incredible gift that day, and my time with her was profound and life-altering in ways I didn't realize right away, but eventually, I learned the significance of that experience and what it meant to my life.

My teenage years were a little more daunting as I grew taller and more awkward. It was not normal for a girl at my age to have a height of over six feet. Some kids gave me horrible looks while other kids felt compelled to vocalize their judgmental opinions. It was amazing the number of kids who did not go out of their way to be friendly simply because I was taller. This was beyond traumatic for me, and it severely affected my self-esteem. I was not a shrinking violet who wanted to hide in the shadows. I truly wanted to be out in the world living life, but I became more withdrawn and always worried what people were thinking about me. I tried to imagine what I would be when I grew up, but I just could not get over my looks and my height, which made it impossible to envision myself being very successful in any field. Still my aunt's words to me about being a nurse resonated within the corners of my mind. I would like to think that if Aunt Blanche had lived, she would be my mentor, guiding me with her wisdom and encouragement. When I considered the idea of becoming a nurse, I believed that anyone could learn the clinical part of nursing, but the necessary nurturing and compassionate qualities did not seem like traits that people could learn. I have always wanted to treat people the way I wanted others to treat me, and innately, caring for other human beings has always made sense to me. As a nurse, I could do something valuable in life that not only fulfills my own passion, but also enables me to give back to others. The nursing profession seemed like the most logical choice and the only career for me.

Having a clear direction in mind, with my plans to become a nurse, I thought college life would be much better than high school. However, to my surprise, it was much worse, because I got sick and spent six weeks at Boston Children's Hospital. Unfortunately, because I was so far behind in my studies, I had to drop out of the University of New Hampshire (UNH) during that time. When I was ready, I started over at Stratham Tech because I was determined to become a nurse.

In 1986, one of my sisters was planning her wedding and her fiancé's mother, Stella, decided that she wanted to play matchmaker. Stella's son had a single friend, named Ron Gauvin, who she thought needed a wife. Stella told him all about my family and let him know about the single and available sisters who might like to go out with him. After hearing her descriptions of us, he decided that he was interested in meeting the tall girl and asked for my name and number.

The idea of someone setting me up with a man was revolting, and I would have preferred to find my own boyfriend in my own time. I was trying to finish my nursing degree and I was not seeking a husband, but she was adamant in her mission to find a wife for Ron Gauvin. I wasn't opposed to the idea of marriage, but it wasn't in my immediate plans for the future. I wanted to be an independent woman first, to ensure that if I chose to marry a man later, it would be an equal partnership because I never wanted to be dependent upon a husband for anything.

Before long, Ron began trying to reach me to no avail. I was busy with my studies and I thought he would give up after a while, but he was relentless in his quest, until he finally reached me. During our first telephone conversation, he told me all about his hobbies, and there were many of them. Then he told me where he lived, what he did for work, and how he had just landed a new job at Hewlett Packard. He was interested in taking pictures of animals, scenery, and he enjoyed his drives up north to go fishing. He was definitely a talker, but I have to admit, I did not have any problems maintaining my end of the dialogue. In fact, to my surprise, I enjoyed our conversation.

Ron seemed passionate about everything in his life, but when he began talking about scuba diving, he sounded positively elated. I hadn't even met him yet, but I could tell that he loved diving more than anything else that he did by the joy in his voice. Ron impressed me with his communications skills and his lack of ego. When he talked about his life, he did not sound self-absorbed about it. Instead, it felt as though he was taking a part of himself and sharing it with me through his eyes. He had a way of drawing me in even though we never met. He asked if I would be interested in learning how to scuba dive. He was so welcoming and I liked that quality in him. Of course, the big test was when I started talking. As I shared details with him about my life, he listened attentively, showing a real interest in what I had to say. I talked about my past, my work, and the pursuit of my nursing degree. I could not believe that our conversation lasted for over thirty minutes, and it ended with us agreeing to meet for a blind date. Of course, blind dates were notorious for being catastrophic in nature, but despite my apprehension, I thought it couldn't be too terrible—not after such a nice telephone conversation.

The evening of our date arrived, January 25, 1986, and it was not the ideal night to go out. The weather was brutal. It was cold, blustery, and snowing outside, which were good enough reasons to cancel, but Ron said he was not letting anything cause him to break our date. I wondered how a man could be so determined to make a date with someone he had never met, and I think that intrigued me even more. While I was getting ready for the date, I started feeling a little nervous. By the time he arrived, my mother answered the door. As he walked in, I stood there with one of my sisters next to me. A feeling of insecurity came over me and I felt compelled to test him. I asked nervously, "Who do you want to take out?" He placed his fingers upon his chin, and he quickly looked around as if he was deciding. Then he looked directly at me, smiled, and said, "Of course, it must be you!" Oh my gosh—I think this guy had me at hello!

During our date, we spent the entire evening talking about everything under the sky—our families, growing up, and our dreams and ambitions. Ron talked about the hobbies he could teach me, and he told me about the places he could take me. Initially, I thought our telephone conversation was too good to be true, but he was even more incredible in person. I never imagined meeting someone like Ron, and I never knew that I could feel so connected to one individual within such a short time. He listened to everything that I had to say while looking at me straight in the eyes. We were actually at a movie theater but the movie was nothing more than a mere interruption in our evening of talking. The saying, "Time flies when you're having fun" was definitely applicable to our evening. I could not believe how quickly time passed during our date.

After we left the movie, Ron drove the long way back to my house, so we could talk more and make plans for the next few days. He was not worried about the snow outside, he just wanted to spend time with me. For the first time in my life, I did not feel awkward or afraid. There was not any doubt in my mind that we would go out again. In fact, we agreed to meet the next morning for breakfast. He even accepted my invitation to attend my family's super bowl Sunday celebration.

Love is a funny thing. You don't really know what it is until it sneaks up on you and captures your heart when you least expect it. I had my doubts and then Ron appeared like a mirage waiting to rescue me from myself. Ron and I continued to see each other every day, never tiring of the other. We eventually began fantasizing about going to Florida together. He was interested in working for a particular diving company in Florida, and if they gave him a contract, he would have a job waiting for him, making our plans possible.

I was going to graduate from nursing school that May and I knew that if we committed to an engagement, I would gladly move to Florida to begin a new life with him. This relationship was beyond anything I could have imagined. I felt so happy being with Ron, and he seemed just as happy to be with me. My life changed completely.

Fitting in did not matter at all because I found someone who could appreciate everything about me unconditionally, which made us the perfect fit.

The time flew by quickly, as Ron and I grew much closer to each other. In fact, by March, Ron and I announced our engagement and began making plans for a December wedding. It was a dream-come-true for both of us. We spent the next couple of months making arrangements and planning our move to Florida. When June arrived, we packed Ron's car and began our trip south. Our move was happening so quickly, and I didn't have a moment to catch my breath or the opportunity to think about everything and everyone I was leaving behind in New Hampshire.

After we arrived, we began to settle in our new home in Florida. Of course, I did not have any regrets because I loved Ron and wanted to be with him, but I have to admit, I needed a little time to adjust to our new way of life. Ron did not waste any time. He immediately got busy working in the office for the dive company waiting for the ideal diving opportunity. The company had promised a dive to a Spanish galleon, and Ron was slated to take underwater photographs of the ruins to recover possible hidden treasures. The diving company owner made many promises to Ron, asking for his patience, as Ron continued to wait for the opportunities that never materialized. Ron needed to continue to earn a real income, but the owner's litany of broken promises placed a huge amount of stress on Ron. This could have strained our relationship, especially because we had not married each other yet, but our bond was strong. We remained a united team throughout every disappointment—our love never wavered.

Ron continued to pursue the big dives but there was never anything available to him. The whole thing seemed bizarre, and even Ron started to notice a few unusual things happening that did not make any sense. As time progressed, Ron figured out that the owner was participating in unethical and illegal practices, which lead to embezzling thousands of dollars from the company. Ron was not willing to compromise his own integrity just to hold onto a job, especially since this job was not generating enough income to pay our bills. He immediately reported what he knew to the FBI. A federal grand jury eventually indicted the owner for fraudulently raising more than $1.4 million. He made false claims to investors about his credentials, and he used their invested funds to misrepresent the value and authenticity of alleged found artifacts to collectors, as a way to lure more investors into his scheme. The authorities learned that most of what the owner claimed about himself was false, making him nothing more than a con artist. This was particularly distressing for Ron because diving was his dream. We came to Florida because the owner led Ron to believe that he had a job waiting with real income. However, that never panned out. Ron felt strongly about doing the right thing and I know that if presented with the same circumstances again, Ron would always make the right choice. I was very proud of him.

Although Ron did not earn much with that company, we still needed that income. Without that job, both of us needed to find other jobs right away to maintain our expenses. We found jobs but we barely made enough money to keep our heads above water. When we sat together in New Hampshire and envisioned our paradise in Florida, this was not it, but we refused to allow this financial setback to destroy our dreams or our wedding plans. We had a lot to do but we managed to put everything together. The happiest day of our life arrived; Ron and I became husband and wife on December 20, 1986. Our day was so beautiful; it was easy to forget the stress of recent events. When we said our vows to each other, we did not know at the time just how meaningful those words would be, but we loved each other profoundly, and we said our vows to each other with only forever in our hearts. There was a reading of a poem during our ceremony, which was perfect for us:

Desiderata by Max Ehrmann

Go placidly amid the noise and haste,
and remember what peace there may be in silence.
As far as possible without surrender
be on good terms with all persons.
Speak your truth quietly and clearly;
and listen to others,
even the dull and the ignorant;
they too have their story.

Avoid loud and aggressive persons,
they are vexations to the spirit.
If you compare yourself with others,
you may become vain and bitter;
for always there will be greater and lesser persons than
yourself.
Enjoy your achievements as well as your plans.

Keep interested in your own career,
however humble;
it is a real possession in the changing fortunes of time.
Exercise caution in your business affairs;
for the world is full of trickery.
But let this not blind you to what virtue there is;
many persons strive for high ideals;
and everywhere life is full of heroism.

Be yourself.
Especially, do not feign affection.
Neither be cynical about love;
for in the face of all aridity and disenchantment
it is as perennial as the grass.

Take kindly the counsel of the years,
gracefully surrendering the things of youth.
Nurture strength of spirit to shield you in sudden
misfortune.
But do not distress yourself with dark imaginings.
Many fears are born of fatigue and loneliness.
Beyond a wholesome discipline,
be gentle with yourself.

You are a child of the universe,
no less than the trees and the stars;
you have a right to be here.
And whether or not it is clear to you,
no doubt the universe is unfolding as it should.

Therefore be at peace with God,
whatever you conceive Him to be,
and whatever your labors and aspirations,
in the noisy confusion of life keep peace with your soul.
With all its sham, drudgery, and broken dreams,
it is still a beautiful world.
Be cheerful.
Strive to be happy.

Although our wedding day was full of happiness and love, we were beginning our new lives together with the weight of the world upon our shoulders. The constant financial worry we shared created more stress than newlyweds should have to endure. Ron felt disheartened by the collapse of the diving company and even more troubled by our fiscal situation. Under the right circumstances, we could have had an income that would have provided us with a comfortable life in Florida. We tried to make it work by being frugal, cutting any necessary corners, and working as many hours as our jobs would allow, but our combined earnings were not enough to make ends meet, and the jobs were not fulfilling for either of us. It was becoming painfully obvious that we needed to make a change before it was too late. Ron and I could talk about anything, and neither of us hid from our problems. We faced our life head-on and discussed the issues that needed the most attention. We spent countless hours talking about our living and work situations, brainstorming, and trying to find a resolution that would make both of us happy while meeting our financial needs. However, the reality of our predicament began to swallow us because no matter how many ways we looked at everything, the results were still the same. We could not find a way to survive in Florida—not with the jobs that were available to us at that time. Going back up north was not what we wanted, but we had to seriously consider packing up and returning to New Hampshire to get back onto our feet. We knew that we would have the moral support of our family and friends, and after the disappointment of not succeeding in our life in Florida, that support was precisely what we needed.

We had already experienced a few loses together, which were difficult and painful for Ron. However, I felt equally hurt in this situation because I had given up everything in my life to move to Florida and begin a new life with Ron as his wife. I remember the ambivalence I initially felt when we moved to Florida because part of me was beyond elated to be with this incredible man, but at the same time, I left behind my friends, family, and previous existence. It took a little time to transition into our new surroundings, and just when I began to feel comfortable and secure with our new life, our Florida dream fell apart.

When we were talking, Ron shared that he had recently lost many friends tragically including his brother during childhood. He said he didn't understand why his reactions to each loss was so different, but figured out that he might have been in denial during these events, while trying to stuff away his emotions as a means of self-preservation. We talked about this in depth, and we discussed the stages of loss and the different ways we handled loss, compared to other people in society. It was comforting to Ron when he began to realize that the reactions he had to those losses were normal. I recognized Ron's sensitive side and I appreciated it. I thought that being able to express his emotions was important, and I encouraged it, especially anger, if he felt it. I believed that expressing anger in a hostile or violent manner was not healthy, but sharing feelings of anger in a calm and constructive way could be quite beneficial. Men during those days often avoided showing emotions because most considered it socially unacceptable, and they interpreted feelings from a man as weakness. What a terrible message to teach men in our society. Whenever Ron expressed himself whether it was a happy, sad, or angry emotion, he always benefited from getting it out of his system. I think this enabled him to communicate much more and it made us an even stronger couple.

We had two weeks left before we were leaving Florida. We tried to make the best out of that time while we packed up our life. During that time, Ron received a call from his family about his nephew who had just committed suicide. Ron was in shock and could not believe the news. As if the sadness for the loss of his nephew was not enough, this situation was even more distressing because Ron wanted to be in New Hampshire with his family, but we could barely afford the move back in two weeks. It was going to be tricky to make a trip home early for the funeral with so little money. Still, we did not have a choice. Ron needed to be there for his family, and we had to make it work.

During our long drive, we shared many thoughts and feelings with each other, trying to make sense of everything we had experienced. We felt a little defeated by the circumstances. I suppose we could have been like many couples starting out who gave up on each other, but Ron and I trusted and loved each other enough that we could find comfort and strength from each other. To this day, our ability to embrace and lean upon each other during so many times of adversity throughout our marriage still amazes me. We knew it would take a little time to get through everything, but we had each other, and we would prevail.

It was 1987, and we had been back in New Hampshire for a few months. It wasn't our Florida paradise, but we were doing much better, and we were together. Ron was getting a job with General Electric, but he needed to take a pre-employment physical first. The results of that exam revealed that Ron was anemic, which turned out to be a side effect from Klinefelter's syndrome. This is a condition occurring in men, who have an extra X chromosome in their cells.

It can affect different stages of their physical, language, and social development, but the most common side effect is infertility, which meant that we would never be able to have children of our own.

Unfortunately, the treatment was an injection of testosterone every fourteen days. As a result, Ron started having painful cramps because his muscles were developing at an accelerated speed from the testosterone. When he asked how to treat the cramps, the doctor suggested that Ron start working out with weights to build his muscles in a healthier and more natural manner. Just as Ron handled any challenge, he rose to the occasion and faced this adversity head-on with determination and commitment, making the best out of a bad situation. Ron immediately began weight lifting and he responded to it with significant endurance. Then, he worked swimming, biking, and running into his workout routine with the goal of participating in a triathlon. Ron adapted well to his new exercise program and started noticing the results. His pain began to dissipate and he was becoming more fit and healthy. I was very proud of Ron for his positive attitude and initiative. Of course, the issue of infertility and children sparked several conversations between us. This was a loss for me, but Ron's immediate reaction was that he felt we were together for a reason, and if children were part of the equation, it would be icing on the cake. Looking back now, I think this was his positive outlook on life, but at the time, I thought he was in denial and unwilling to face the loss. I suppose if he was not willing to face it, he would not have been willing to join an infertility support group with me, but he did. I think it helped both of us significantly because we were able to discuss and process all of our feelings regarding the loss of children in our lives, as well as the other losses we had experienced. We tried to be aware of our reactions and allowed ourselves to grieve those losses throughout all of the stages to enable us to move forward and not allow it to overwhelm us. It was not easy, but our love was clearly the foundation that held us together and enabled us to face the challenging issues in our life. Participating in a support group was so much better than sweeping our emotions under the rug and hoping for the best because that would never have worked out very well. Being part of a group like that helped us to work on our own issues and support others in the same situation because we witnessed many couples who fell apart after letting infertility come between them. Ron and I could easily understand how it happened to other couples, but we promised each other that we would never let infertility or any other issue come between us. Nothing was more important than the love we had for each other.

Ron and I began making plans for our future as we envisioned our lives without children. We talked about the many ways our marriage would be happy and full because of our love for each other and all of the things that we were going to do together. Ron's optimism was infectious, and it was impossible not to see the glass as being half-full.

Ron started teaching me how to fish and canoe. He was at home in the water, whether it was an ocean, lake, or pond. We had so much fun together, and it was entertaining at times. When he started showing me different aspects of photography, it was incredible to see how he viewed the objects that he wanted to capture. He saw beauty in the most unlikely places and helped me to see that same beauty through his eyes. He was passionate about all of his hobbies, and he was extremely patient in the way he taught me.

Ron made everything appear to be so effortless and inviting, which made it more enjoyable. Even baiting a fishing hook or using a favorite lure was fun and always a guaranteed laugh. If I didn't understand something, he took the time to explain it so I would understand without making me feel inadequate. I couldn't wait to learn and do more because I really enjoyed doing these activities with Ron.

In June of 1991, Ron's father received a diagnosis of the advanced stages of prostate cancer. I had just graduated from UNH with my Bachelor's degree in nursing. Between my training and the information I received from some physicians, it was important that I explained the reality of this cancer to Ron so he understood his father's prognosis. At that time, a few treatment options were available, but the results of a bone scan showed a positive reading, indicating that the cancer was in Ray's bones. This was not very good news. Sadly, this meant that Ron's father probably had less than a few years to live.

Ray Gauvin was a strong man, and despite his prognosis, he chose to continue working to get his full retirement from the navy yard. I think Ray wanted to make sure his wife would have as much as he could provide while he was still alive to make things easier if he did not make it.

It seemed as though every time we began to let our guard down to get comfortable, another loss appeared. Ron and I spent many hours talking about his father's condition and Ron's reaction to this shocking news. I wanted to do anything I could to help Ron cope so I began researching to find documentation that would help both of us. Throughout this process and all of the materials we read, we started understanding the need for a positive attitude, especially when facing loss. It seemed like such a simple way of thinking and hard for me to understand why I did not figure this out on my own. Of course,

I learned that if we are spending all of our time and energy focusing upon the negative aspects of life, and if we are asking ourselves, "What if the worst thing happens," then we will not have much time or energy left to focus upon, "What if the best thing happens." Wow, it cannot be that simple but it is. We will ourselves into some of our own doom and gloom, and it is a proven fact that stress can affect us negatively on a physical level. People who are fit, healthy, and eat right have strokes and heart attacks because they allow stress to overwhelm their lives. Why wouldn't we choose to remain calm, relinquish fear, and focus upon hope? How can we find a strategy to succeed in anything if we continue to view the glass as being half-empty? This was quite a learning experience for Ron and me, and I think this was the beginning of a new way of looking at life. I don't think I realized how important this awareness was at that time, but it became extremely relevant to our lives a little later.

Ron loved scuba diving so much and he wanted us to share the beauty of it together, so he encouraged me to learn how to scuba dive. This gave us the opportunity to refocus our energy on something more productive, rather than wallow in anguish over the circumstances that we could not control. We needed to grab life and embrace it together. I was happy to learn because I wanted to see and feel what Ron experienced when he went underwater. Ron was a great teacher, and while he wanted to share the fun and beautiful parts of scuba diving with me, he always stressed the importance of safety. He never took any risks while teaching me; he did everything by the book. He showed me how to breathe properly, and he always checked to make sure I was comfortable and that I could use the equipment with ease.

We took our first dives of the year in late June to prepare for our vacation at Martha's Vineyard in July. As I became more comfortable, we started doing night dives together—diving to depths of ninety feet. This was our goal so that we could do boat dives while we were on vacation. The experience was amazing.

After coming off one of those dives, Ron complained about having some middle ear pressure. I never remembered him having any trouble before so this was a bit unusual. Initially, I thought his eardrum might have been damaged, which could be painful, but this seemed to be much worse.

His ear pain persisted over the next couple of days, and it began to affect his balance, almost like having vertigo. His condition did not improve, and he started to walk into things and lose his balance at work. Ron's coworkers went with him to the infirmary where he explained the sequence of events leading to that point to the doctor. He also told the infirmary nurse about his dad's condition and thought it might just be stress from that situation. The infirmary doctor sent Ron to an (ENT) ear, nose, and throat specialist. Ron followed up on this appointment right away because he did not want to miss any of our vacation in Martha's Vineyard, and he was looking forward to the diving that we planned. Imagine Ron's disappointment when the ENT sent Ron for an MRI and then advised him not to dive while we were on vacation, just in case. Ron was disappointed about the diving, but he was still excited about Martha's Vineyard with me. They did the MRI, and then we left for our vacation. We were both a little concerned about the results, but we kept that in the back of our minds. Our primary goal was to relax, enjoy the ocean, and enjoy each other.

We did our best to distract ourselves, but we continued to wonder about the issue with Ron's dizziness and ear pain, and we could not help but talk about it. Without knowing what was wrong, we could only speculate, which would never give us accurate answers to our questions.

Our time on Gay Head Beach was the most inspiring, with the clay cliffs behind us and the sound of the ocean waves all around us. This helped us to relax and feel energized at the same time. There was something soothing and magical about this beach, and we felt so lucky to be there. Ron told me that after being in such a beautiful place with me, no matter what the results were of the MRI, he would now have the strength to deal with it. Ron may not have been able to go scuba diving, but somehow, he felt a strong connection to his spirituality on this trip, and that seemed to fulfill him even more.

Ron was facing two possibilities that the ENT had proposed—multiple sclerosis (MS) or an acoustic neuroma, which was a benign tumor of the nerve that connects the ear to the brain. Neither were good options, but Ron had a stronger fear of multiple sclerosis. He witnessed the slow deterioration of a good friend who had MS, and he could not imagine living like that. Ron thought that a benign brain tumor was removable and his chances might be better. I'm not sure that Ron was being as realistic about the situation as he could have been, and I thought that maybe he was stuffing away his emotions. Of course, since then, I've learned a lot about my husband and the way he copes with life's unexpected curve balls. His positive attitude was probably more helpful to him and us then than I could have realized. While I was worried about Ron and the uncertainty of his health, he was worried about making sure we enjoyed our time together. He said we could worry about the results of the MRI after we returned from vacation.

When we got home, the answering machine had several messages on it. Two were from a neurologist that had seen the results of the MRI. The tone of her messages had a sense of urgency as she requested Ron to make an appointment for Monday. This alarmed Ron, wondering what could be so important. We also had a message from the ENT himself, with instructions to call on Monday. I am not sure what I was feeling after hearing those messages. I wanted to be positive for Ron, but in my experience, doctors did not usually act with such urgency unless it was something major.

In Sickness and in Health

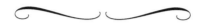

Monday morning finally arrived. Ron called the doctor's office to make an appointment. When he got off the telephone, I could see by the expression on his face that something was wrong. Ron told me that Dr. Pinto-Lord wanted him to come into her office immediately. I felt a little nauseous because I knew that a doctor would not request an immediate meeting unless there was a serious issue to discuss. Ron pulled me close to him, hugged me, and said, "We'll get through this together." How did he do that? How was he able to find so much optimism in the face of so much uncertainty? I should have been the one comforting Ron with positive reinforcement, but instead of focusing upon himself, he chose to be reassuring to me.

We did not waste any time. We gathered ourselves and headed straight to the doctor's office. During the drive, we talked the entire way, remembering the bliss of our vacation and the hawks flying above, while we were lying on Gay Head Beach. I think we were both trying to find solace in the peace and serenity that we felt during our time away. In our eyes, the hawks represented flawless nature, beauty, and life. We felt that they were a symbol that would provide us with the strength we needed to face whatever was awaiting our arrival. As we continued reminiscing during our drive, Ron suddenly saw a hawk in the sky, and said, "There it is, we'll need him." I wanted to believe in that hawk the way Ron did, but I felt the fear creeping into me.

When we arrived at the doctor's office, the receptionist handed Ron a ton of forms to fill out because he was a new patient, and they needed his complete medical history for their own records. The whole thing seemed a bit overwhelming for Ron so he handed the paperwork to me. He relied on my help to explain the questions to him while he gave the appropriate answers to me. One of the questions stopped me in my tracks, asking if the patient had any previous seizures. Ron's response was no, but I couldn't help but remember an incident several months prior when I found him on the bathroom floor having what I thought was a seizure. Of course, when I described it to the doctor who treated Ron at that time, the doctor ruled it out. I didn't have any reason to doubt the doctor's expertise so I put that thought out of my mind. However, reading the question on the form made me wonder. The fact is that seizures are not identical in nature and affect people differently, both neurologically and physically. Some people convulse, flail their arms, fall, shake, or foam at the mouth while experiencing a seizure. Others may not exhibit any obvious outward physical symptoms at all. Those individuals may only feel it internally while experiencing a memory lapse, loss of speech, or mass confusion.

Thinking back to that moment, perhaps there was more to the incident with Ron than we thought. Maybe I was too eager to accept the doctor's answer as gospel, without exploring it more or maybe I was in denial willing to accept the answer that I wanted to hear. Either way, I was beginning to learn an important lesson regarding the vulnerability of our healthcare system. With everything that happened to Ron along the way that led to that moment in the doctor's office, I began putting the pieces of an unsettling puzzle together in my mind. I felt a huge pit growing within my stomach, and for the first time, I was truly afraid for Ron and for us.

Shortly after I finished filling out all of the paperwork, the receptionist called us into Dr. Pinto-Lord's office. As we entered, she greeted both of us with a handshake, but then she muttered to herself, "How did I end up with these MRI films?" She looked a little perplexed as she pointed to the MRI films clipped to the light box on the wall. She did not say anything to us initially while she studied the image of Ron's brain. Then, she asked me to share the sequence of events leading up to that point. I began to explain Ron's symptoms and everything that had happened. Being a nurse, I was familiar with the structure of the brain as seen on MRI films, which made it difficult for me to focus on what I was saying, because I could not help but glance over at the light box. Then, while I was speaking, something caught my eye, which distracted me from what I was telling the doctor, and I stopped in mid sentence. I realized that I saw something did not belong. I immediately pointed to the films and asked the doctor, "That does not belong there—what is it?" She calmly responded with clarity, "It is a tumor in the middle of the temporal lobe of his brain about the size of a walnut." I think my entire body froze in horror, and I wasn't entirely sure that I heard her correctly. I thought she had just said that my husband had a brain tumor, but I did not know what to say.

When I looked over at Ron, expecting to see some kind of a reaction on his face, he smiled and said proudly, "My wife is a nurse." What—did he hear what the doctor just said? Dr. Pinto-Lord just gave the most distressing news about his health, but his face was blank. I didn't know what was more shocking—the news of this brain tumor or my husband's response to it. Instead of responding to what she said, he bragged about me being a nurse because I spotted the tumor. He seemed so calm and disconnected at that moment as if we were discussing another patient. I wanted to scream, but I quickly realized that I needed to maintain my composure for my husband. I did not understand his reaction, or in this case, his lack of reaction, but I knew that I could not be there for him if I was falling apart.

Dr. Pinto-Lord continued explaining the details of Ron's tumor, its position on his brain, the potential symptoms, and the risks that this tumor imposed. Ron continued to remain calm as he listened to everything she was saying. I noticed that he kept glancing over at the large white area of the tumor on the MRI films because I was doing the exact same thing. I remember wondering what Ron was feeling during those moments—was he sad, afraid, or angry? I also wondered what the doctor was thinking while having to discuss something so serious. Unlike many doctors who slam their patients with bad news and subsequently walk out, she did not rush the process. Dr. Pinto-Lord took her time and explained everything in specific detail to make sure we had a full understanding of Ron's condition.

Perhaps Ron was in shock or in denial, but thinking about it now, I believe he was a billboard of courage during a time when he would have been justified in showing extreme sadness and fear. A million things go through your mind at once when you hear a doctor describe the brain tumor that has invaded the one you love. It is almost impossible to decipher one thought from the other because of the sheer shock and disbelief. When this affects somebody you care about, loss suddenly becomes a real possibility. You just cannot imagine the pain and fear that person must be feeling, hearing that he or she has a brain tumor. Watching it happen almost feels like a hazy dream with life suddenly flipping into slow motion, while you desperately try to catch it and change it back to the way it should be. Except, you can never get there in time, and when you wake up, everything is exactly the same.

It was surreal and just as difficult trying to wrap my mind around the unimaginable. What kind of wife would I have been if Ron looked over at me and saw a death sentence stamped upon my face? Those first few moments were the most pivotal in this journey because he needed me—his wife and life partner to believe in him and let it be okay for him to hope. Did I consider what this meant for my life? Was it selfish of me to entertain thoughts about my own existence, knowing that my husband must be living his own personal nightmare? Selfish or not, I could not help but wonder what this meant for us as a married couple. I knew what having a brain tumor generally meant for a patient, and I knew that a treatment plan would be the next step. Would Ron have to stop working? Would we be able pay our bills? Would our health insurance cover all of his medical costs? I had many things to consider. However, those thoughts had to live in silence for the time being while I tried to be as strong and supportive as I could for Ron.

The doctor continued discussing everything with us for about an hour, and she made sure that she addressed any questions we had before ending the meeting. When we left Dr. Pinto-Lord's office, we had an appointment for Ron to stay overnight at the hospital to get an electroencephalogram (EEG), to test him for any seizure activity. He also needed an arteriogram, which was an X-ray type of test to visualize the blood vessels in his brain. These tests would give the doctor a clearer picture of Ron's brain and the tumor, to determine the best treatment plan.

Maybe we needed a second opinion. Wasn't that something that people normally did with such a serious diagnosis? Dr. Pinto-Lord seemed like a perfectly competent doctor, but doctors made mistakes all of the time. Perhaps another doctor would have a more radical plan that would ensure Ron's recovery. I wondered if I should have urged Ron to follow up with a second opinion, but I was a nurse. The truth was that nothing could change what I saw on those films. I did not need to be a doctor to know that her diagnosis was spot on, and that the next logical step would be to have the tests that she ordered.

As we walked out of the building, I felt drained and exhausted. It was as though a huge truck had plowed both of us over. We were in shock because the entire world had changed for both of us in a matter of seconds. My husband had a brain tumor, and this was the first time as a nurse when I felt completely useless. I wasn't sure what to say to Ron to help comfort him, but then he did not act like a man who needed comforting. Instead, he just held me while we stood in the parking lot in disbelief. At that moment, I thought he might let his guard down, and he did a little with some tears, but he remained calm through those emotions and said, "Remember our favorite song while we were in Florida, 'when the going gets tough, the tough get going.' I'm going to be all right, and at least, it isn't MS." Ron had initially worried that he might have multiple sclerosis (MS) because of its degenerative nature, and he felt relieved that he didn't have it. Maybe he still thought as he did before that his brain tumor was removable. I guess Ron's behavior should not have surprised me. He was always the one who went out of his way to make others feel better and to find the silver lining, but I am still worried about his reaction while he stood there comforting me. I think he was contemplating his plan of attack, ready to defeat this alien intruder within his brain. Thinking of how Ron always approached the challenges he faced in life with his various sporting events—maybe this was the only way he could deal with having a brain tumor, except this would be the biggest challenge of Ron's life.

When we got home, I spent some time going over everything that Dr. Pinto-Lord had told us during our visit with her. She stressed the importance of being a wife to Ron as opposed to being his nurse. I thought I could be both because I could use my knowledge and background to help Ron through treatment and explain things that he did not know. I believed that my profession would give him an advantage in his care that he otherwise might not have had. Then again, I understood the doctor's point because Ron needed the emotional support that only a wife could give, especially with so much uncertainty ahead. The odd thing is that when Dr. Pinto-Lord seemed surprised to receive Ron's MRI films during our first meeting, it was because she happened to be on call when the radiologist saw the results. It was by pure chance that the films landed in her possession. Dr. Pinto-Lord's professionalism, bedside manner, and knowledge were comforting compared to other doctors I had worked with recently. She seemed to have an appropriate balance between the level of detachment that doctors need and the compassion that patients and their family members need. She was forthright and she did not hide the severity of the tumor, but she handled it with the right amount of sensitivity. I appreciated this along with her explanation to Ron about the tests that he would need to take. As much as I wanted to assume the nursing role by explaining these tests to Ron in more detail to prepare him, I followed the doctor's advice, and I chose to talk to my husband like a wife and discuss what we were thinking and feeling along with our concerns. Dr. Pinto-Lord was right, Ron needed my love and support much more than he needed a nurse to repeat what the doctors were going to explain to him.

Ron and I talked as we always did about everything happening at that point—his feelings, my feelings, and our fears. Ron had already faced loss in his life, but this represented much more because his brain tumor brought mortality right to our front door. Ron and I wanted to be realistic, and we felt it was important to talk about the various stages of grief while we tried to figure out how we were going to cope with this diagnosis. I considered myself a strong individual, but I was not sure if I would be strong enough to maintain the positive attitude that Ron needed. I felt selfish and guilty at times for even thinking of my own fears, knowing what Ron was facing, but I made every effort to stifle those fears as much as possible for his sake.

We realized that we could not sit on this information alone for too long. We needed to inform Ron's parents, but Ron knew that it would be too difficult to tell them in person. Instead, he called and explained everything over the telephone. It was all he could do to remain calm and not cry as he listened to his mother cry. The only thing he could do to console her was to show his mother that he was optimistic to avoid projecting any of his fears onto her. Ron continued to reassure and comfort his mother as they talked, and he continually repeated to her, "I'll be okay."

Despite everything that occurred that horrible day, life had not stopped. We still had bills to pay, and we could not ignore the rest of our responsibilities. That night, we both went to work as usual—only this time, we found ourselves sharing the news with our friends and coworkers. I remember talking about our vacation and thinking how it seemed like a lifetime ago. For me, telling other people about Ron's brain tumor made it feel more real and difficult to pretend away. I think the toughest part was seeing the expressions on their faces after saying that Ron had a brain tumor—some with sympathy, some with shock, and others with sadness—as they immediately viewed this as Ron's death sentence. Of course, most made encouraging comments, promising to pray for Ron and for us, while others remained silent as they did not have the courage to say what they were really thinking. I would like to say that it got easier each time we spoke about it, but that isn't true. There wasn't anything easy about this situation, and not knowing what the future held, left me in a constant state of fear. Ron did not show it, but I knew he had to be feeling it, and because he kept his emotions in check, I found my internal numbing switch to be the rock that I thought he would eventually need. We still shed some tears from time to time, but neither of us fell apart.

Dr. Pinto-Lord had explained that due to the location of the tumor and the suspected type, it was probably slow growing, and we could take the time we needed to make any necessary arrangements for the procedures. Both of us took time off from work because it usually took a few days after the arteriogram to recover, and I wanted to be with him the entire time. Of course, knowing that the procedures were scheduled and quickly approaching, we needed to update the remaining members of our families. Considering how difficult it was on the telephone the first time with Ron's mother, it was apparent that we would have to do the same with the other relatives because talking to them in person would be more than either of us could handle.

As we made the calls, Ron spoke to his various relatives initially, and he explained as much as he could about the situation until they began asking too many questions that he could not answer. Whenever that happened, Ron handed the phone to me. I can't say that it was any easier for me because I struggled between sharing my fears with them and trying to remain strong for Ron as he stood by listening.

After Ron had the procedures, the EEG results indicated he was having seizure activity, and it was probable that the incident a few months prior was in fact a seizure. This further reinforced my thoughts that as a family member, I needed to be an advocate for Ron, which meant questioning a doctor's opinion when warranted. I couldn't help but think that had we known it was a seizure back then, perhaps we would have a better handle of the situation.

The arteriogram results determined that the tumor did not have a blood supply going toward it and it had been there a long time, which confirmed that it was slow growing.

According to the doctor, these test results were good news but not definitive. She also told us that she was requesting a neurosurgery consult because they needed to do a biopsy—a minor surgical procedure removing cells to determine the pathology, type, and grade of the tumor, which would enable them to recommend an appropriate treatment plan. They graded the tumors on a scale from one to four in relation to the tumor's speed of growth—one being the slowest and four being the fastest and the worst. Ron trusted me implicitly, and he was completely reliant upon my decisions at that point, but I was reliant upon the neurologist's recommendations to help me make those decisions. It was difficult to know the right thing to do for Ron because the doctors could only offer the clinical options available to us along with the risks and benefits. I could never be sure I was making a decision because I was his wife or because of my medical knowledge. All I could do was trust my instincts as much as possible and pray that I would do right by my husband.

When we tried to set up a time for the biopsy, the local neurosurgeon declined to do the procedure. He was concerned about the tumor's location, and he did not want to risk causing Ron further harm during a biopsy procedure if anything went wrong. He recommended sending us to Boston where he felt we would find more equipped doctors who could take the risk with better chances of success. This was a little frustrating because we wanted to get Ron's treatment as soon as possible. Having to go to Boston to see yet another doctor would only delay the process more. Ron asked, "Who was the best?" They responded by giving us a list of the most reputable neurosurgeons in Boston. With Dr. Pinto-Lord's assistance, we chose the best neurosurgeon on that list. It seemed like such an arduous process, with entirely too much back-and-forth, to get Ron the treatment he needed. It was long and exhausting, but through it all, Ron was calm and hopeful. When we discussed how afraid I was, Ron shed a few tears. I knew it was hard for him because he wanted to take care of me, but he needed to focus on the next step, which he was ready to take. Ron felt inspired by a book we had recently read by Bernie Siegel called "Love Medicine and Miracles." It was about maintaining a positive attitude and that miracles happen to patients every day. Ron carried those thoughts with him as he moved forward.

The following Monday after work, Ron was beyond exhausted. He had told his story several times to friends and coworkers—none quite believing that he was even at work with a brain tumor. I think he needed to share this with the people around him to bring it to reality, to validate his experience, and to know that they cared about him and were in his corner. I wondered if he saw the looks of fear on any of their faces and, if so, how did he feel about it.

The following week seemed like an eternity as we waited for our scheduled visit in Boston to arrive. The anxiety of not knowing the next sequence of events was overwhelming, causing many sleepless nights and tears. If we had moved from one phase to the next, it would not have been as difficult as the waiting that we had to

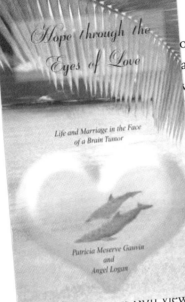

ors, tests, and procedures. Ron had to get
and Women's Hospital in Boston because
vn assessments based on the most current
ot to mention, hospitals preferred doing
if they had been done at other facilities,
:urrent information but also for liability

he intrigued Ron along with the fact that
ed it. I noticed the logo on the magnet,
oring good things to life." The other
when we saw hawks flying around again
-what were the chances of that happening
... won viewed it as a good sign, and I did too.

After the MRI, we found our way to the neurosurgeon's office. We sat in the waiting room until the doctor was ready for us. While we waited, Ron noticed the other people in the room with us who had shaved heads and scars on their scalps. He said, "I'm not the only one you know." He recognized and respected that he was not the only person going through this type of experience. I think knowing that helped him to realize that he was not alone in what he was experiencing. Ron could have been absorbed in his own anguish, but I could see that he felt genuine empathy for them, as if they were in their own private club that no one else in the world could understand. We sat in amazement watching several people in lab coats scurrying around the office and exam rooms. Ron and I were both curious and wondered if any of them would be meeting with us. They seemed to follow each other one by one as Ron said, "Yeah, like a bunch of ants, in and out of each of the exam rooms." This became our little joke and amusement while dealing with the anxiety of waiting. I felt overwhelmed by the lack of control I had with the situation at hand, but I gained some semblance of relief by making light of the situation. Humor was a great coping mechanism for us as a distraction from stress.

Finally, the receptionist escorted us into an exam room. Of course, it was more of the same endless waiting. You would think the serious nature of a brain tumor would have rendered a more expedient response.

Then later, the door opened and four men walked in. Only Dr. Loeffler introduced himself to us. When I looked at his nametag, it read "Radiation Oncologist." He was not a person that I was ready to meet. He briefly scanned through Ron's folder of information, and then he stated, "Not the right type of tumor." Just like that, the four men blew through the door like a whirlwind. Ron and I both started laughing from sheer nervousness. Ron said, "Must not be the right kind of ant food." We laughed until the door opened again.

This man's nametag read, "Dr. Peter McL. Black, Neurosurgery." He entered the exam room alone and extended his hand to Ron first, and then to me. As he sat down on an exam stool, his calming presence was a relief compared to the frenzy of other doctors who had just been there. He asked Ron several questions regarding all of the events that had occurred to that point. Then the doctor performed a neurological exam. Ron asked, "Can you find out what this thing is in my head?" Dr. Black proceeded to explain the biopsy procedure. Of course, the only three details that Ron seemed to remember that Dr. Black said were the words "a halo, awake, and home the next day." The meeting with Dr. Black was less than five minutes long and created days of questions, sleepless nights, and preparation for the surgery scheduled two weeks later. He seemed to know his stuff, but he did not take the time with us that Dr. Pinto-Lord did on our initial visit, and it was a little disconcerting. Still he was supposed to be the best, and I had to rely upon that.

Ron was going to be wearing a halo device, which was a type of head frame that they used to position the head precisely for tumor location and to prevent the head from moving during the procedure. In addition, they were going to extract the cell sample from the tumor while keeping him awake. Then he would return home the following day. Ron rehearsed these details verbally many times over the following few days, as he shared the itinerary with family and friends. He talked about everything with confidence, which even reassured me that he would be okay. This was just another example of how Ron chose to comfort and reassure everyone else despite everything he was facing. However, our conversation the night before the surgery was less confident and more anxiety filled as we discussed what Ron wanted me to do if he did not wake up. The idea of considering the worst-case scenario was frightening enough, but we were willing to face our fears. We knew that the most responsible thing that we could do was discuss the possible end-of-life issues that we did not want to discuss. We went over what Ron would want regarding code status and burial if anything happened to him. Of course, we were organized and realistic with our conversation about the things we knew could happen, but we did not have the slightest clue what we were going to endure over the days following his surgery.

When the day of Ron's biopsy arrived, they escorted him to pre-op an hour early, which made him a little nervous. It did not help that he heard a CAT scan technician say that they needed to hurry because the surgeons were waiting for him. I think the last thing that anyone with a brain tumor would want to hear is that they are in a hurry when they are about to cut open your head. A little part of me felt a twinge of anxiety too, but I pushed it deep within me to be as positive as I could.

The process of applying the halo was the most painful procedure Ron had every experienced. Even though they gave him an intravenous line with a medication that was supposed to help relax him, the enormity of the pain from attaching the halo while screwing the bolts into his scalp caused him to go unconscious. My only hope was that they gave him amnesia-inducing drugs to prevent him from remembering that pain.

The helplessness I felt while waiting was tremendous as I sat crying and wondering if I had helped Ron to make the wrong decision. Again, I was learning what it meant to be an advocate. Imagine if the patient did not have a family member or spouse to help make decisions and speak with the doctors. It was a difficult position for me to be in because Ron really trusted my judgment. I wanted to do all of the right things for Ron to give him the best chances possible. My mind was plagued with doubts, wondering if we were too eager to have the biopsy done. There was a reason why the other neurosurgeon refused to do this procedure—what if he was right? What if the tumor's position made the risk too high? What would other doctors have decided to do under the same circumstances? Was Dr. Black really the best neurosurgeon available and would he do the procedure himself or subject Ron to inexperienced medical students just learning? Over the next several hours, I asked myself an array of questions, second-guessing every decision I had made. I tried to distract myself by reading, pacing, eating, and doing needlepoint while I sat in the family waiting area.

The four hours waiting seemed like an eternity, and then finally, Dr. Black called me. He said that they needed to observe Ron in ICU for a while, but I could go in and see him. I felt such a sense of relief. When I went into ICU, Ron was awake, but his eyes could not focus on me. Maybe he just needed a minute to acclimate after such a grueling procedure, but then I noticed other things. He had slurred speech, his right arm was extremely weak, and he could barely move his right leg off the stretcher. I expected him to be exhausted and maybe a little disoriented from passing out, but I did not expect any of this. "I'll be okay," he said to me as I tried to hold back my tears. Over the next hour, his condition fluctuated; and the doctors said that by morning, they would repeat the CAT scan to check for any bleeding that might have occurred during the procedure. I hated to leave him, but he needed to rest after all of that. I prayed that his condition would improve.

I arrived the next morning at the hospital and rode the elevator up to the tenth floor. I noticed Dr. Loeffler among the twenty other people on the elevator. He recognized me and enthusiastically said, "Your husband is doing well—he has a great tumor." Seriously, he actually just said that my husband had a great tumor. I could not believe my ears and I was so angry that I blurted out, "What do you mean—he's paralyzed!" The doctor didn't offer any explanation or response at all; he simply got off the elevator when our floor arrived and left me standing there puzzled. As I walked down the hall, I had a few minutes to think about the doctor's remark and then I thought that maybe I overreacted. Perhaps the doctor had already examined Ron that morning and everything was back to normal. That would have explained it.

I started to feel hopeful again, expecting the nightmare of the previous evening to be gone, but that was not the case at all. Ron did not have any movement in his right arm or right leg. This was supposed to be a simple procedure—a small extraction to test the tumor—that is all. Why did the biopsy go so horribly wrong and why did the doctor think everything was okay, when clearly it was not?

During the next four days in the hospital, Ron showed a glimmer of his strength and determination. He reminded me that it would be his attitude that would get him through this. Ron must have been afraid, but he didn't show fear, he showed nothing but courage. The doctors that paraded through his room said that he should get stronger over the next few months. They did not offer much of an explanation beyond that. The doctors did say that the biopsy results indicated the tumor was a grade 2 or 3 anaplastic astrocytoma—a good tumor. This was a lesson in brain tumor terminology from Dr. Black that would be mine to share with hundreds of inquiries over the next few months and years.

All tumors in the brain are potentially malignant or deadly, but benign tumors have an incorrect label because if they are not treated, they are also deadly. The grading system for gliomas received their name for the type of cell, which they grow and divide. An anaplastic astrocytoma is a slow growing glioma tumor that invades the brain in a star shape with fingers growing like the points into the brain. The grading is ranked from II to IV with a stage IV being the rapid growing tumor. I did some research that indicated that the two-year survival rate was 50 percent among patients with anaplastic astrocytomas as compared to the 5 percent among those with glioblastomas. In another study, the median survival was twenty-seven months in patients with anaplastic astrocytomas and eight months in patients with glioblastomas. With these kinds of numbers, I refused to look at that information as anything other than statistics based on a controlled number of people, which was a helpful coping mechanism for me. I did not intend to lump Ron into one category of patients that did not necessarily apply to him. I guess I took a more logical approach with this situation while Ron used humor as his coping mechanism—choosing to lighten situations with laughter—probably to keep from shedding the tears.

Ron did not need treatment for his tumor at that time because of its slow growing nature, but he needed extensive therapy because of the weakness on his right side that resulted from his biopsy procedure. Without hesitation, I requested the hospital to release him so I could bring him home with me, because I knew that we could get nursing and therapy home services. His doctors recommended Ron going into a rehabilitation facility to build his strength, but Ron pleaded with me to take him home and not make him go into rehab. My instincts told me that I needed to take him home because Ron would do much better at home with me. I didn't think he would benefit from the stress he would feel being in a place where he absolutely did not want to be. Not to mention, I had started a new job as a nurse in a home health agency a few weeks prior, and I had told Ron the benefits of home care over rehabilitation. Ron listened and knew he would get great care and would feel much more comfortable in his own surroundings.

Ron never doubted his own determination. The therapist came to visit three days a week, and Ron worked extremely hard during those sessions as well as on his own the other days of the week. Giving up was not even a consideration. In fact, the therapist often complained that Ron was working them too hard, but his hard work paid off because within six months, he regained all of his strength and his speech improved.

We learned to accept Ron's condition and live with the circumstances that surrounded it, but he had to watch me struggle with the mounting bills, the denied applications, and the re-applications for social security disability, along with the threat of no health insurance, and then the introduction into vocational rehabilitation. The pressure I felt continued to grow because the weight of the world seemed to be upon me. Ron could not return to his job because of the machinery, and he could not drive for a year because of his seizure medication. There wasn't a manual available showing how to deal with all of the problems that we faced after his hospitalization. Any of these issues individually would be an enormous strain on any person, but combined, and then compounded with a brain tumor diagnosis was beyond character building. Still, these issues were a total distraction at times from thinking and talking about the next stage of Ron's treatment.

Through vocation rehabilitation, Ron was able to continue school. In a psychology class, he wrote a paper describing the stages of grief through his experience of this recent hospitalization. He entitled it, "Why Me, But Why Not Me." This paper was a therapeutic way for Ron to acknowledge and process his feelings through this experience and to learn the meaning of acceptance. Ron and I could talk about anything, and we did from the moment of our first telephone conversation until now, but I think that when an individual puts his or her feelings down on paper, the pen unlocks a door that reveals the deepest thoughts and emotions that we often don't share, even with the people closest to us. Ron wrote:

"Every time somebody hears the word tumor, the first thing that comes to his or her mind is death. It's bad enough to have a tumor in any part of the body but the brain. That area controls our every emotion. When we think of laughing, there is a signal sent from neurons within the brain to the muscles around the mouth, and we laugh.

"When my wife would say, 'God, I hope that there is nothing serious,' I would say something like, 'Don't worry, Pat. I'm sure it's not bad. I can handle this.'

"I'm used to seeing doctors because I can feel a broke leg, arm, or a sprained knee. These are all areas where I can feel that something is wrong, but I cannot feel this. I can't even begin to see it.

"I would think to myself, You are healthy. You are a person preparing for triathlons. You are running, swimming and bike racing. I am supposed to do everything. The world is in the palm of my hand, or is it? I feel so good, there can't be anything wrong—not me. Why me? I did not do anything wrong.

"I was admitted to Wentworth Douglas Hospital on August 1, 1991. The doctors said that they wanted to do several tests to see if the tumor was being fed blood by new growing arteries. I had several test an arteriogram, which determines the location of any arteries in relation to the tumor, and a CAT scan, which generates a photograph of the precise location of the tumor, and finally an EEG, which is for determining if I am having electronic seizures. Throughout all these tests, I would still say that nothing is wrong."

Reading how Ron expressed himself made me wonder if other men in his position could have been as brave and forthright with their emotions as he was in this paper. He wasn't just sharing his experiences with me; he was opening himself up to others, and it made me extremely proud of him. Ron also wrote:

> "I had the usual bargaining. I would often say, 'Why me, God? What did I do?' I would say, 'I'll go to church more often—honest I will.' I'll try and not swear. What can I do to change this? I would ask help from all those loved ones that are gone. I just would say, 'Why me, God? Why me? What did I do?'

> "I would feel depressed knowing my wife is working so hard to make the money that we need. Yet when she comes home, she has to face the way that I am. I cannot write to help her with the bills—she has to do it all.

> "I felt like an outcast one time at the camp. The children saw me with my head shaved with stitches, and I could barely balance enough to even sit down. I had a quad cane to assist me with walking, but I still needed help. I don't hold that against any child. They are too young to understand. They feel sorrow in their little way.

> "I have come to accept the way that I am. I can not change it. I can't even bargain to improve it. We all have our misfortunes, some worse than others. I live each day the best way that I can. I spend time with my friends, family, and my beautiful wife. These people are the ones who gave me the strength to go on.

> "There are a lot of obstacles up ahead. I do not know if I will regain all that I have lost. I do not know if I will have difficulty in achieving my degree. I do not know if I will scuba dive, bike race, or ever run again.

> "I am labeled disabled. What is disabled? It is just a word. We are all disabled in one way or another. It actually means that you are different.

"It is sad to believe that I may someday die of this tumor. I thought that I was really healthy, but we are all going to die someday. To what—God only knows. As long as we do the best that we possibly can for every day that we are here on this earth, we can truly achieve what it is that we want out of life.

"Each morning, as I awaken and smell the air, I give thanks. This is one more day that I have to give it my best. This is one more day I can be with my friends, family, and wife. These are more important to me than any amount of money or that time can bring."

My husband's words touched my heart in ways I can never begin to explain. He described denial, bargaining, and acceptance; but what I read was courage—courage to face the unthinkable, courage to share his private thoughts, and courage to truly feel in the face of the worst and most uncertain kind of adversity.

For Better or for Worse

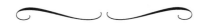

Ron had to have an MRI every three to six months to monitor the size of his tumor. It was beyond challenging to live between these appointments and the ever-increasing expenses that fell upon us, but we decided that despite the bills, we needed to think about something other than the MRI appointments. To nurture our spirits a bit, we scheduled a windjammer cruise in the West Indies to celebrate our fifth wedding anniversary. I did not realize how desperately we needed this time to ourselves. For one week, we escaped from our life's mayhem and forgot about all of our problems.

After we returned home, it was time for another MRI. As we waited to see Dr. Black, the door opened and in walked Dr. Loeffler, Radiation-Oncologist. I asked, "Why are you here?" He proceeded to let us know that his specialized radiation treatment was available at Brigham and Woman's Hospital in Boston and that he has been anxious to get Ron started on it. Ron was going to be the eighteenth patient in this protocol, and with the location of Ron's tumor, it would be an ideal modality.

The details of this treatment were overwhelming at the time, but we dealt with each issue individually, which Ron conquered as each surfaced. Some of these issues included the need to miss school for the thirty treatments. Ron wasn't happy about this, and he was concerned about how it would affect his classes, but he spoke with his instructors and found that they were all quite understanding and flexible, advising Ron to concentrate on his treatments. Another problem was the transportation issue. Ron needed a way to get to his treatments, which was challenging, because I could not always be there. Fortunately, I called C&J Transportation and shared our dilemma with them. They responded with thirty free bus passes from Dover to Boston's South Station where Ron could take the subway *T* the rest of the way to the hospital. He had never taken the *T* in Boston before, and the switching from one train to the other was a little confusing as it would have been for anyone who had never used the public subway system. Ron worried that he might get lost, but together, we practiced the trip a few times for his first few treatments to make Ron feel more comfortable and familiar with the stops and changes. Then, he did it on his own for the remainder of the treatments.

Ron remembered the halo, and he was adamant that he would not have another halo applied. They reassured Ron and fitted him for a different head frame device that they mounted by a mouthpiece. This new device was also an experimental process called "Relocatable Immobilization for SRT." Stereotactic Radiation Therapy (SRT) required the technology of radiosurgery, including sophisticated treatment planning systems, high-energy therapeutic machinery, and stereostatic immobilization devices.

With thirty trips on Ron's itinerary, he needed some inspiration. He recorded a song that they could play while he was receiving the treatment. He chose Pat Benatar's "Hit me with your best shot." He also sat in the children's waiting area rather than the adult area because he found that the children had similar courage. He found that he gained strength not to complain because if the children and their parents could get through it, he could too. He met the parents and facilitated one mother to ask to see her child's 3-D MRI image. Ron had asked and thought it was helpful to have an image of the shape, size, and location of his tumor making it a real entity that he was confronting.

This outreach and attitude was the beginning stages of Ron's transcendence. He was not going to be defeated. The courage that he displayed was inspiring to others. He truly felt that this treatment would not slow him down. Despite knowing that a major side effect of radiation was tiredness, he did not miss a day and insisted that we take another trip to the West Indies at the end of his treatments.

Ron had accepted this diagnosis and he was ready to live with the tumor. He had to remind me that we needed to get on with our lives. Unfortunately, his dad was getting worse so our focus shifted to him. Ron recognized and acknowledged that his dad was not dealing with his diagnosis. Ron wanted to help his dad deal with the illness and get through it. He and his dad spent a lot of time fishing together. They often headed out early in the morning, having planned a day ahead of time, even placing the canoe on the truck the evening before.

As his dad's condition deteriorated, they devised easier alternate ways to carry the canoe. Ron paddled more and more on each trip, and he said that they didn't talk very much while they were on these fishing adventures. Ron realized that they didn't need to because it was quality time together. Ron admitted during that summer of 1993 that it would probably be his last year to fish with his father.

Before Ron's father died, he told us that he hoped that he was dying so that perhaps Ron would not have to suffer. When we asked Ray what he meant, he said that he was content with the way Ron was dealing with his illness, and he was proud of how strong Ron had been and would continue to get with this tumor. I think that Ray Gauvin believed that if he died, God would spare Ron's life.

I was able to help the family keep Dad at home until his death, but we were only able to get hospice care for him during the last two weeks of his life. The family would not speak about the inevitable until the end. They were sad and they did not want to accept it. Ron and I had our own private conversations and supported each other through the end. Ron was the only person that publicly cried during the funeral service. Uncomfortable with his display of emotion, they escorted Ron out of the funeral home. This shocked me beyond belief. I could not understand his family's response to Ron's emotions or the reasons why they felt compelled to hide their own grief. I spoke to Ron about this unusual reaction for a long time after the funeral; it just did not make any sense.

This loss resulted in us examining where we were going within our own lives. Ron continued to attend school, and I pursued some management courses through my job. During one of the courses, I had to write out some goals for my career. Consistent through my five-year, one-year, and six-month goals, I wanted to start a brain tumor support group. I had not discussed this with Ron, but it was apparent that he would need to be involved in this next plan. When I brought it up to him, he was on board with my ideas. We started researching the best way to run a support group. We didn't want to start this project without having a strong understanding of the process to ensure that our group would be beneficial to all involved.

In the fall of 1994, Ron started noticing more difficulty with the strength of his right arm and leg again. His right side peripheral vision was getting worse too. We wondered if the tumor was coming back despite all of those radiation treatments. We went back to Boston for a new MRI to figure out what was happening. After having a repeat Spect scan, which was a more specialized MRI, they determined that fluid had been accumulating in the area of the tumor. These cystic sacs needed draining, and the plan was to leave the drain in for future use.

As before, the scheduled surgery was to be an overnight stay, enabling Ron to come home the next day. Having heard this, I just could not believe that they would let him go home in less than twenty-four hours after doing a draining procedure on his brain. Attempting to maintain our sense of humor about it, I bought Ron a card that showed a guy with his head in a drive-up window like

McDonald's. The caption read, "Drive-through Brain Surgery." Amazingly, it was true. Ron went into surgery in the late afternoon while they kept him awake. They used the modified halo device, as promised, and they gave him an amnesic medication so he would not remember. Ron claimed that he remembered everything including when they pushed the drain into the cyst. I couldn't even imagine what that must have felt like. Before I made it to his room the next morning, they had already discharged him. Although the weakness on his right side was not any worse, it wasn't any better either. Consequently, I requested outpatient therapy for Ron.

A few years prior, I worked with a neurological-psychologist who specialized in head injury rehabilitation. This individual was the manager of a day treatment program. They provided transportation and a full day of occupational, physical, and speech therapy. This was the ideal outpatient facility for Ron. In a short time, the care manager, therapists, and doctors all became friends with Ron, and they were supportive of his goal to work someday. This group of therapists convinced Ron to get involved with the other clients as well as the Northeast Passage organization. Northeast Passage was a nonprofit group that encouraged disabled people to reintroduce themselves to outdoor activities. Ron joined the group to help them with fund-raising, and he raised the most money for the year, winning a trip to Nantucket.

Ron never allowed the spotlight to be on him at any point during his participation. He always looked for ways to be helpful to others. By socializing with other people during therapy, he learned that while he had many issues to face, there were others dealing with more. Ron's philosophy was to make the best of any situation. I have to admit, his way of thinking was contagious to everyone around him. He encouraged other patients and staff, and when they discharged Ron from the program, they threw him a party. I think that Ron benefited greatly from this organization, not only from the staff, but also from the other patients.

In 1996, Ron had to have surgery again, to drain more cystic fluid that accumulated around his tumor. We handled this surgery with amazing strength and courage, having gone through it before. We felt confidence and respect for the doctors along with the other medical professionals. I had asked all of them as many questions as I needed to feel supported. They were always happy to answer and they took the time to make sure I understood. I was comfortable with the process of pre-admission, and I knew how to reach the doctor during and/or after surgery. I felt enlightened and I was ready to share this knowledge with others. Even during Ron's surgery, I spoke with other family members about my plans to start a support group, and they seemed to be in my corner.

In preparation for the support group, I attended a one-day Bernie Siegel workshop, the "Psychology of Illness and the Art of Healing." I had read many chapters of Bernie Siegel's recently released book, "Peace, Love and Healing," aloud to Ron, which helped Ron to maintain a positive attitude throughout his treatment. In addition, Dr. Siegel's first book helped me immensely when Ron first received his brain tumor diagnosis. I felt extremely excited to be at the workshop because I knew that I would gain valuable information that could help me even more in my life with Ron. I did not shy away when I had the chance to meet Dr. Siegel, and while he signed my copies, I shared some of my story with him.

Bernie Siegel was a pediatric and general surgeon from Connecticut. After he retired, he began writing books and conducting support groups with the goal to help people suffering with chronic and tragic illness. He had a different way of helping people to face their illnesses with a more positive outlook while using love and hope to help with the healing process. During this workshop, Bernie asked the group of over three-hundred people, "How do you know if you are enlightened?" Then, he asked, "If I was to take you to dinner, what would you tell the waitress you wanted?" I stated loudly, "Lobster." He asked me to stand and said, "I know this woman's story, and if you go home today without meeting her, you have missed out on meeting an enlightened person." The workshop was incredible and I was thrilled to be part of it. I could not wait to tell Ron what had happened. This experience was the beginning of the self-realization that I had coped with our situation well. Ron's positive attitude and strength had been so pervasive that I was coping with issues at a different level from what I had realized.

Our experiences with Ron's most recent hospitalization had been another indication of how much our coping skills had improved, and we were eager to share our growth with others. After contacting several other support groups and different brain tumor societies and foundations, Ron and I decided that we were ready to start the support group we had discussed previously. We found several in Massachusetts, but we could not find any others in the New Hampshire area. We attended a group in Burlington, Massachusetts to find out some details and to get a few tips from the facilitator. Then, we contacted the New Hampshire Brain Injury Association and attended their support group to learn as much as we could for Ron's benefit and for our own research. At that point, we felt as though we had prepared enough to start our group. In addition, we found the ideal facility to house our support group—everything was falling into place.

After Ron's discharge from his outpatient therapy, he volunteered at a local hospital to develop work skills. Vocational rehabilitation had determined that he was not employable through a neurological-psychological evaluation. This neurological-psychologist's insistence of this had halted any hope that Ron would be able to receive assistance for job placement. During that evaluation, the doctor told Ron that he should not stress himself with the idea of work and that he must be depressed. On top of that, the neurological-psychologist told me that I was in denial because I didn't realize that Ron's tumor was progressing and that I should accept that Ron was dying.

This was when I realized just how important it was to be Ron's advocate. He needed someone to cheer him on, believe in him, and to understand him enough to pick-up where medical professionals leave off. It was so easy for a doctor who barely knew Ron to write him off as a lost cause. He placed Ron into the same category of every patient he probably treated before, and he was ready to dismiss Ron's life as being over. Then, he thought it was appropriate to suggest the same to me. In my opinion, his attitude and assessment was not only wrong, but it was unprofessional. As a family member, we must be there for our loved ones when they are under the charge of a healthcare facility. Doctors do make mistakes, they are often rushed, and they rarely have the time or the inclination to become acquainted with their patients. How can a doctor truly assess the recovery potential of an individual without knowing his or her full history—not just the medical history, but also the personal history? It is a proven fact that many people have survived well beyond the bleakest clinical prognosis, against all of the odds, without any medical data to support the miraculous results. Maybe it is a higher level of consciousness, divine intervention, will to live, or sheer hope. Regardless of the explanation after everything we had faced, I learned that we must fight for our loved ones especially when they don't have the energy to fight for themselves, unless or until they say otherwise.

I was so angry by the neurological-psychologist's inaccurate assessment of Ron; I immediately called Boston to find out if he had heard something that Ron and I had not been privy to from the last surgery results. Dr. Black in Boston reassured us that we knew everything about Ron's condition, and there was not anything new to concern us. What right did the neurological-psychologist have to give me such a grim prognosis when he was not the one treating Ron, and he had not been part of the years of hard work that Ron put forth for his recovery? Telling me that I should give up on my husband because he was dying was not only erroneous—it was reprehensible. Not to mention, I requested this evaluation because it was the criteria that the vocational rehabilitation needed to formulate their plan for Ron.

I felt helpless because I had not fully realized how much we were at the mercy of our healthcare professionals until then. As a nurse, I learned to trust the word of every doctor as being the expert who had the authority to make life-altering decisions regarding their patient's healthcare and overall well-being. This was a huge awakening for me because clearly, infallibility in doctors did not exist. I did not lose faith in the healthcare system, but I gained a better understanding regarding the need for patient advocacy. This was an important point that I had planned to share in our support group.

Ron refused to give up on his goal of returning to work so we sought advice from another neurological-psychologist who advised us to do three things. First, he said that Ron should try a volunteer position for a period of six to nine months to demonstrate his job skills. Second, he said that Ron should start speech therapy to document progress in his cognitive skills. The third suggestion was to obtain an independent neurological-psychologist evaluation.

We followed the advice while feeling hopeful. The volunteer work and speech therapy process was simple, but to convince the vocational rehabilitation to accept an external neurological-psychologist's evaluation was a challenge.

The anger and frustration from this most recent experience motivated us to continue with our support group plans and launch it. We knew that we could offer a comfortable and safe forum for people in our position to gain mutual support and understanding. We expected to learn as much as we were prepared to share. At our first meeting, eight people attended. Sometimes we had as few as three attend, and as many as fifteen, at our subsequent meetings. There was a little structure, which made the informal nature of the group more inviting and comfortable. The discussions varied from meeting to meeting, and the participants took turns opening up with the other group members. Ron shared his story and compared notes with others regarding his treatment and surgery experiences. Ron also received the attention of a newspaper reporter who wrote a story about Ron, our life, and our support group. We were happy to gain the publicity. This was an incredible networking experience, and through all of our associations in and out of the group, we developed a common bond that probably gave us more support than what we gave to them. We were so grateful for the opportunity.

Month after month, we recognized that we might need to deal with the loss of some of our members. Others in the group were dealing with tumors that were more aggressive. As their conditions had deteriorated, they attended less frequently, and eventually, we received a phone call from family members sharing that they had died. That was probably the most heartbreaking part of the experience. Over a Christmas holiday break, three of our members died. As the group leaders, we felt compelled to help the remaining group members cope with these losses, which turned out to be more than I could handle.

Ron was handling it much better than I was, but he was sad because we had created our own special family with that group, and it was painful to lose any of them—never mind three within the same time frame. Many questions came from our family and friends who wondered the reason why we wanted to do something so depressing. I thought we were doing a good thing for others that would ultimately be therapeutic for Ron. Was this support group too much for Ron to handle? At times, I had my doubts, but a friend gave me Ashley Prend's phone number. She was a licensed psychotherapist and grief counselor who authored several books regarding loss, grief, and self-awareness. When I called her and explained my situation, she offered to give our group a gratis appearance and speak about her areas of expertise to inspire our members. I read her book *Transcending Loss* in preparation for the event, and I met with her ahead of time to discuss the details of her book and how her philosophy applied to us. We discussed the connection of dealing with a brain tumor diagnosis and the losses that occur. She realized that we were not like the support group members who were dealing with the loss of other members. Although we were coping with those losses, we were also facing the adversity of an illness within a marriage.

Ashley's willingness to talk to me about the issues surrounding my life with Ron was so helpful and inspiring. We also discussed how Ron and I had been applying her book's philosophy to our grieving process regarding the losses we had faced along our journey. I confirmed with her where I thought we had been, and she agreed that we were well on our way through transcendence. I appreciated her time, guidance, and support. When she spoke to the group, there was an opportunity for open discussion regarding the people who had died. This enabled the group to acknowledge and honor the deaths as well as the survivor's illnesses.

I was starting to realize that our reactions to our life's adversity and the length of time we had dealt with it had been different from other's experiences. I wondered if we could find a commonality with any other long-term survivors. I would soon receive an answer to my question.

Through contacts with the folks in Boston and the Brain Tumor Society, I received an invitation to lead a panel discussion for long-term survivors for the annual meeting/symposium. This was an incredible opportunity, which I truly appreciated. I interviewed each of the five members of the panel and discovered a common thread that ran through all of their stories. None of them allowed the brain tumor diagnosis to control their lives. Amazingly, they were not afraid to make long-term plans and talk about the future, and they had a real love for life. These survivors were beyond transcendence as Ashley described in her book, which was truly inspiring.

Ron continued to pursue the possibility of working, but the only barrier remaining was his inability to drive. He was unable to use his right arm and his right leg was weaker. Armed with a nine-month record of volunteering, along with a speech therapist report, we approached vocational rehabilitation again and told them that we wanted a driving evaluation. I think we had reached enlightenment because I wasn't just asking for "lobster" this time. I did all of the necessary research regarding the process of these evaluations, the names of the individuals who conducted them, and the cost. We walked in prepared to present Ron's very detailed plan. With a lot of hesitation, they approved Ron for driving, and within a few months, he was back on the road with an adapted vehicle. They agreed that the prior neuro-psych evaluation was flawed. This was a huge victory!

The next step was to find a job. The vocational rehabilitation center assigned a job coach to us who worked with Ron for over a month with success. By the fall of 1997, Ron was back to work—another triumph—after so many disappointments throughout the years. We were finally heading into the right direction, and Ron was elated that he could work again. Because each paycheck was precious, Ron declined the use of automatic deposit. He wanted to cash his checks and see the fruits of his labor within his own hands. Ron was quite fortunate to be working with a great group of individuals who appreciated him and who felt inspired by his attitude and determination.

In early 1998, things took a turn for the worse. Ron's speech increasingly became worse. He had difficulty with specific areas of speech and language such as the inability to say nouns. I noticed that this happened more when he was tired. I struggled between positive thinking and denial because I hated that this was happening to him again. Because I was so worried, we made another trip into Boston for yet another MRI. It was déjà vu for us as we scheduled another surgery. This disappointed Ron because he had just started working again. He was feeling so good about himself because he was able to do something productive that contributed to our lives, and he had found some of the independence that he had lost for a while. Ron was afraid that his downtime would cause him to lose the job that he had worked so long and hard to achieve.

The surgery appeared to be successful and delayed the deterioration of his speech for a little while. In addition, he only missed one month of work. Unfortunately, that delay was brief as Ron's speech began to decline more, making it difficult to communicate. During the fall of 1998, Ron's boss realized that it was too difficult to converse with him regarding work-related issues, which ultimately affected his performance. Ron agreed to leave his job in October. I contacted his job coach on several occasions to mediate and to provide support, but in the end, leaving was actually a relief to Ron. He adjusted quickly to life at home again, and he was content to help with the housework and care for our dog.

Getting back to speech therapy was a necessity, but unfortunately, the therapy did not help Ron this time—his speech continually declined. To make matters worse, Ron had to show signs of progress for the speech therapist to justify providing service to him according to their policy, but he wasn't improving at all. This was discouraging and frustrating on so many levels especially because Ron started having difficulty communicating with me. I was always Ron's safe place to fall, but without the ability to articulate his fears to me, I can only imagine how much this frightened him. Ron's condition continued to worsen throughout 1999.

By February 2000, we had entered into a new century as well as a new world of growing technology. With Ron's continual speech deterioration, we had to schedule another surgery to drain more cystic fluid from his brain. However, because of the advances in medical technology, a new option became available to Ron. Instead of just draining the fluid from the cysts, the surgeon could safely perform a craniotomy and clear out the cysts that were growing from the tumor, making this the most aggressive type of surgery. The incision on his head started from one spot over his left ear and ended in the middle of his scalp.

Ron was nervous, but he was confident that the doctors in Boston would do their best. While we were hopeful that he might regain some of his speech, we were also aware that there was a chance that Ron could lose the remaining function of his right hand because of this surgery. Ron did not dwell on the things that could go wrong. Instead, he chose to focus all of his energy on being positive, expecting only the best results.

After Ron came out of his surgery, there was only a minimal change in his speech as well as the function of his right hand, even with some therapy. The reality of Ron's speech never returning had been a difficult loss to face and process. I could not imagine how we would communicate with each other effectively, which felt impossible at times. Not knowing his thoughts and feelings was even more devastating to me. How could I help my husband cope if he could not express himself to me? We could always share our feelings with each other, but that was not going to be an option anymore. I was feeling so discouraged by our situation until a friend gave me a glimmer of hope and introduced me to a man who taught visual-gestural communication. He described how people could communicate through facial expressions, hand gestures, and body language. Then, he explained that as husband and wife, we had already developed our own special form of communication, and we could speak to each other in several more ways than we had even realized. Reflecting on this, I felt reassured and I started to notice the numerous ways we communicated daily—ways that I had taken for granted. I knew when Ron was upset, sad, tired, excited, or appreciative, and I knew when he was expressing his love for me without even saying a word. Wow, I should have figured this out on my own, but because verbal speech was our regular form of communication, it made sense that I didn't realize it until someone pointed it out.

It would have been easy for me to sit around and wallow in self-pity for my husband's losses, for my losses, and for the married life that we would never have. It has been so hard because I love Ron with every fiber of my being, but the reality is that the marriage we both envisioned disappeared the day the doctor told us that he had a brain tumor. Still, despite the myriad of challenges and losses that have invaded our lives, we have enjoyed many blissful moments together before and after the diagnosis. Knowing that visual-gestural communication was a viable option for us, I was optimistic that we would find more blissful moments waiting around the corner.

For Richer or for Poorer

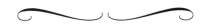

How can we predict the life that we will have after joining in marriage? Our lives are no longer just our own. Every decision we make has a strong bearing on the life of the other—our career choices, income, and expenses. It is one thing to consider the normal household budget—rent or mortgage, utilities, insurance, etc. However, when medical bills pile on top of your regular household expenses, everything else feels the impact.

It was difficult for me to solidify any career, having to take care of my husband. He needed my attention day and night, and I was the only one who could effectively communicate with him. Hiring an outside nurse would have been more financially challenging, and I did not believe that another nurse would treat him with the same love and care that I had given him all along.

Therefore, I had to figure out how to make a career work well enough to meet our financial needs and still enable me to meet my husband's caregiving needs. This was a challenge as most jobs were not conducive to our situation. To make matters worse, I had to have a hysterectomy in 1997. One of the difficulties in caring for another human being was finding time to take care of myself. Whenever I felt anything that seemed off, I usually ignored it or told myself that my nursing background was enough to handle any possible health issues. The truth was that I did not have the time to worry about eating properly, exercising, watching my weight, or any of the other number of issues that resulted along the way. Ron's sterility early on in our marriage ended the possibility of having children of our own. When he received his brain tumor diagnosis, having children through any means, biologically or through adoption, was not an option anymore. However, knowing that in my mind did not change the loss I felt from having a hysterectomy. I suppose that my way of thinking stemmed from not having the control over my own body and life. It was one thing to decide that I could not give birth because of Ron's circumstances, but another to see an integral part of my body disappear forever, taking away some of my womanhood. Thirty-six wasn't that old, but suddenly, I felt aged. I had to take pills that older women took, and I think that experience changed my life forever. I did not fight it, and I was prepared to move on to the next phase of my life, but as with any loss, it took a moment to accept.

I had worked as an intake coordinator for a local Visiting Nurse Association, and I had various nursing-related jobs before that. Eventually, I changed jobs to a position at a home health and hospice service. I was in charge of education and compliance as well as clinical operations. This was a good job with better pay, but it was still challenging to pay bills and be there for Ron as he needed. I also took a part-time job as a hospice nurse. I think my real job was juggling as I had several balls in the air, trying to balance my professional life with my life at home. My work was necessary to pay the bills, but Ron needed me more and more as time progressed. It was daunting trying to focus on the needs of the agency staff and hospice patients with my constant worry about Ron being home without me. Yet I felt extremely comfortable in the hospice work setting. I loved being able to care for people especially those at the end of their lives in hospice. I wanted to help make their dying dignified to let them know that they were more than just patients or bodies. I believed in my work, but I felt pulled apart. The harsh reality was that Ron could not work anymore. Consequently, he had to receive social security disability for income. While the monthly disability payments helped a little, Ron was dependent upon me financially because we could not survive on his disability earnings alone. His monthly income equaled what many people earned in only one week, and that was being generous. As long as I continued working, I had full benefits, which we needed for his healthcare.

Fortunately, my career changed in the fall of 2000 when I started working in the home health software industry as a clinical implementation specialist. My dream was to travel throughout the US and make a few trips abroad. Then, after a year, I hoped that the company would promote me to a management position. The trips I made consisted of trade shows and onsite training for supervisors.

With the growth of the home health industry and the expanding population of seniors, this field had become more prevalent. The demand for point of service documentation had also expanded, and my company had their thumbs on the pulse of change to update their software and keep up with the industry and the demand of regulations.

I had developed training material incorporating the most recent changes in regulations. I spoke at several workshops and provided onsite training. With that experience, I hoped that the company would ask me to present at the NAHC convention regarding the cost savings and motivations of utilizing the latest technology in home health.

Ron had been able to travel with me throughout the US, which actually eased the stress of my out-of-state work. Before, I had to worry about what he was doing at home alone, if he was comfortable and safe, and if he needed anything. Traveling with me solved that problem because I could see him every day and limit his time alone when I was working. We not only stayed in the implementation sites, but we also explored those areas. As a result, we discovered many beautiful places within the US.

Ron's health remained stable, and he was able to communicate really well using visual-gestural communication, along with a nonelectronic version of an augmentative communication device. This nonelectronic version used a series of pictures that he pointed to when he needed to indicate a place or item not in the immediate area. He also became proficient at drawing pictures of the things that he wanted to communicate as his artistic ability had remained unaffected.

Many probably thought I was insane for pursuing my Master's of Science in Management degree at Antioch New England Graduate School, with everything I had on my plate. At times, I questioned my own sanity, but my job was extremely fulfilling, it paid the bills, and I knew the degree would make my transition into management a natural progression, going from my home health agency eight-to-five job to a stronger position placing point-of-care devices within the hands of clinicians. I learned about changing organizations, management, strategic management, project management, and of course my thesis—Ron's autobiography. Writing about his life gave me an opportunity to reflect upon our experiences together, to share Ron's life and the lessons we had both learned, how we both had survived his brain tumor, and the realization that even this was not enough of a barrier to prevent me from following my passion. I wanted to travel and I wanted to make sure that Ron had a full life. Although financially it was not feasible to have him come with me on all of my trips away, he was able to see many special places.

This job was an answer to countless prayers. I was eager to learn as much as I could to grow and to give something back on a variety of levels. I always had an interest in computers, and this was the ideal way to help others. I truly admired the commitment and genuine concern that this company had for the entire organization within as well as their clients.

The truth is that I could have stopped, and then blamed Ron's situation from holding me back. However, through a lot of soul-searching and some strategic planning, I realized that pursuing my career dreams would benefit both of us.

While I was cultivating my career, I realized that my desire to live in Florida near the beach was strong. Actually, the ideal arrangement would be for us to live part-time in both places, enabling us to enjoy our little piece of paradise and still have quality time with our families.

I had a heart-to-heart talk with my mother about what I was feeling. I explained the reasons why we wanted to split our time between Florida and New Hampshire. We wanted to be able to live part-time in both places. I discussed my initial desire to live in Florida with my mom, and in her infinite wisdom, she suggested that we do a short-term rental in Florida. I knew that she didn't really want me to be that far away from her, but at the same time, she understood the enormous pressure I felt by our life and all of my responsibilities. My mother also understood how much Florida meant to both of us. I had something to consider with her suggestion. I wanted her advice about other areas of our life too. We had sold our home and moved into a manufactured home. We thought that this move would lower our costs, and eventually we could move to Florida again.

Ron and I had many things to consider if we were going to make this move, and we had to figure out how to make it work financially. Because my job was flexible and remote, I could work from anywhere and not worry about our location. We had a little money saved because we had previously sold Ron's truck when he had to stop driving. There were still a million unanswered questions, and the fear of the unknown was overwhelming. Logistically speaking, we could not commit to a big move like this unless we had a plan with a clear vision in mind. We could not just pack our bags and go without knowing for sure what was awaiting our arrival. That was okay in the beginning of our relationship because we were younger.

Even then, we didn't do very well in Florida as two healthy people, full of incredible dreams.

The more I explored the idea of moving back to Florida, the less sense it made. There were so many obstacles in our way, and Ron had enough hurdles to overcome already. All of his doctors were in Boston, and it would be too difficult to establish that same trust and rapport with new doctors in Florida. I just did not see how we could make it work. I think I was finally ready to give up the idea to focus upon our home in New Hampshire.

Then, one Sunday afternoon during a moment of serendipity on a flight to New York City from Boston, a man boarded the plane and took a seat in my row. There were several empty seats nearby, but he chose to sit right next to me. I didn't mind because I was doing my own thing—needlepoint. I especially enjoyed doing needlepoint during flights because it was relaxing, and it gave me a chance to do something recreational that I didn't usually have enough time to do at home. The man noticed my needlepoint and began talking about it. Because our seats were so close together, I worried that it might have been disruptive to him, so I apologized in advance. He didn't feel bothered by it at all. In fact, he said that he enjoyed doing needlepoint too, which was surprising. I hadn't known any men interested in doing those kinds of crafts.

We started chatting about all sorts of things, and then he shared his experiences from September 11, working for the port authority. Oddly, I had been in the city that day too so I felt a kinship with him as we discussed how those tragic events affected our lives.

The man continued about how he was feeling burnt out by the high demands of his job along with the hustle and bustle of the city, and he wanted to leave New York to move to Florida. After having spent so much time thinking and talking about Florida, it was a little strange running into a stranger who had plans to move to Florida—what an unusual coincidence.

It seemed that his goal was to move there by the end of the year. In addition, he described the house he was building. He mentioned that he had originally planned all of this long before 9-11, but his previous plans had not materialized. Then, after such a life-altering event, he realized that life was short and he needed to just do it.

Between the conversation I had with my mother and my encounter with the man during my flight—I could not help but notice a common thread connecting my recent interactions. Was this a coincidence or was the universe sending me a message?

The man and I parted ways after passing through the baggage claim. As with many airplane encounters, I knew that I would never see him again, but our conversation sparked something in me, and I found myself daydreaming about Florida again, thinking how Ron and I could actually do the same thing. I was beginning to feel confused. I wanted to do the responsible thing and make the best choices for Ron that would benefit him the most, but every time I've veered away from the idea of Florida, something has drawn me back into that thought process. I know Ron's heart and I knew if asked, he would say that he wanted to go there to live. Ron wasn't the one I needed to convince. My internal struggle made this a point of contention because I could not base any of my decision-making upon the desire to live in Florida. If it was that easy, I wouldn't have felt so conflicted. The only way we could live in Florida is if I could be sure that we would succeed there. With everything on my plate in caring for my husband, I couldn't be sure that I could live with the same level of security in Florida that I was experiencing in New Hampshire.

Later, after arriving at the Brooklyn Marriot, I decided to go for my first walk across the Brooklyn Bridge. This was exciting because I had always wanted to see New York City from the bridge's vantage point. The weather was finally warm enough to enjoy the outdoors so rather than unpacking, I left my luggage in the room and I went for my walk. It was such a nice day, and I was really enjoying myself. Of course, halfway across the bridge, I stopped and I called my mother to do the usual "guess where I am." I did this often with her whenever I had visited some place new or interesting. The fact that I could call my mother on that "cell thing in your pocket" as she put it, amazed her, and she got a huge kick out of my calls.

The view was spectacular and I wanted to share that with her. I described everything I saw, trying not to leave out any details. If Mom could not be there, then I wanted her to enjoy the experience vicariously through me. When we finished our conversation, I turned around and headed back toward Brooklyn. I enjoyed looking at New York's skyline and all of the people on the bridge. There were so many people out who clearly had some place to go. Just as I approached the end of the bridge, I heard a car honking its horn. Don't get me wrong, a honking horn in New York City was a regular daily occurrence, but this particular horn caught my attention because it seemed a bit obnoxious. When I looked over at the car and its driver, he appeared to be waving a badge at me. I moved my head to get a clearer view, and I realized that the driver of that car was the same man who sat next to me on the plane. What were the chances of that happening? I think the hair on the back of my neck stood straight up and I had goose bumps all over. New York City was far too large for such a random coincidence; I came to the realization that the universe had to be sending me a clear message. My mother initially suggested it, and indirectly, so did this mysterious man who enjoyed needlepoint. Ron wanted to go and admittedly, I wanted to go to Florida too. I felt a huge sense of contentment and relief because maybe it was time for Ron and me to return to our paradise in Florida. We never wanted to leave the first time, but our circumstances at the time were beyond our control. I knew that Ron would love this idea, and being near the ocean would make him extremely happy.

I didn't waste any time making a plan for a winter rental in Florida as a trial move. I figured out everything that we would need to do or finish in New Hampshire, and I made a list of things to do upon our arrival. Six months later, we were on a flight to Pensacola, Florida to look at winter rentals on the beaches of Navarre. I'm not sure of the reason why, but I had a habit of encountering people on the planes who had valuable information to share. During our flight to Florida, we spoke to a man who had traveled all over the world. He told us about different places in Florida, and he said the best beaches he had ever seen were between Pensacola and Navarre. This was precisely what I wanted to hear. When we arrived in Florida, we picked up a car and we took a drive along the national seashore to Navarre Beach. We parked in a beach side parking area and walked on a footbridge that crossed over the sand dunes. The man on the plane was right about the beach; we saw the most spectacular site we had ever seen with pure white sand and clear emerald water. Suddenly, the details that worried me before did not seem so important. I cried because I knew we had found our home. The sites that we discovered while we were there were unimaginable. Dolphins were playing in the surf, and we saw several sand dollars within the sand. Our walk along the beach was beyond invigorating, relaxing, and breathtaking. Having put so much time and thought into this, I had the opportunity to feel the weight of the move, unlike the first time we moved to Florida. We were going to move away from family and friends, enjoy a life of no snow, or frigid weather, and the opportunity to have family visit us. Florida was our dream-come-true once again, and we knew we could make it work the second time.

After we stayed in Navarre for our first winter, it didn't take long before we purchased our home and made this a more permanent transition. We initially rented our new house to the sellers while they finished building their new home. In fact, we had to delay moving into our house because of Hurricane Ivan, which directly hit our area in September 2004. The house that our tenants were building was on the water and needed repairs from the damage caused by the hurricane, delaying their move by two months.

Once we finally moved in, everything felt so much better. Ron loved living in Florida in our new home, and he did not have a single complaint, but it was difficult for me to watch him struggle to walk on the sand of the beach. He didn't have any walking issues when we were here the first time, but the weakness in his right leg affected his balance and ability to walk through certain areas of the sand that were harder to navigate. He also had moments of difficulty trying to get up from the sand chair. The sand often sifted under his feet when he tried to get up, making it hard to gain the leverage that he needed without slipping. My heart ached for him because living in Florida was his dream, but he could not enjoy every aspect of it as he did before because of his illness and physical limitations. However, he refused to allow his disability to take away the happiness he felt being there next to the ocean. If he could deal, then so could I, and we would just have to improvise and be more selective about the areas of beach where we wanted to walk so he could still enjoy it.

These walks were good exercise for both of us. I had been successful at losing weight through Weight Watchers. However, maintaining it was a different story. I didn't have a definitive exercise routine, which made it difficult to keep the weight off. The frustrating part for me was that I not only had to keep track of my own point system and food intake, but I had to keep track of Ron's as well because he was following the diet too. I had to record each food item for him and for me, which became confusing at times. I tried to make the best of the situation because I thought his willingness to work on his weight was a good thing.

In addition to taking better care of ourselves, we were trying to bring more friends into our lives. One of the shocking things I've experienced is hearing and seeing the reactions from existing friends and extended relatives regarding Ron's condition. So many are actually amazed that he is still alive today. I've reached a point now that when anyone asks how he is doing, I tend to be a little cautious and selective about my response, not giving too many details. Some days are good days, and some are not. The worst part is when he has just had a seizure because the last person in the world I want to tell is his mother. A mother's love for her child, even her grown children is different from any other love. I try to avoid sharing too many of my concerns or feelings right before an impending surgery. I'm sure she has enough of her own worries, without me compounding her stress with mine. Sadly, we had friends along the way who chose to cease their associations with us. It is difficult to make new friends when Ron cannot communicate with others or go out with the guys for a night out.

I must say that we have some very nice friends and neighbors in the area who do not feel intimidated by Ron's disabilities. In fact, they have developed a picture-drawing system as a tool to facilitate communication between Ron and them. It can be extremely difficult, but they continue to persist and make an effort to understand the pictures he draws. Of course, it is a little funny when I walk into the room because more often than not, I can look into his notebook at his drawings and know precisely what he was trying to say.

One of our friends in the neighborhood moved away a few years ago, and it has been difficult for Ron to communicate with the remaining neighbors. Ron's method of communicating by drawing pictures was helpful in conveying what he was trying to say. He seemed to be better at writing numbers, but when he attempted to articulate words, they were not exact. I could usually figure it out. For instance, whenever he wanted to indicate a number of weeks, he couldn't process the information in his mind well enough to say four weeks or one month. However, if he said, "Monday, Monday, Monday, Monday," that indicated four weeks—the number of weeks he wanted to convey. If he wants to say any given day of the week, he usually doesn't have any difficulty saying that day correctly after saying the days leading up to the day he wants, "Monday, Tuesday, Wednesday, Thursday." It took some time to figure out his process because I'm sure it was difficult for Ron to assess his own process, given the complexity of his brain function. However, I've found that if I exercise patience with him and let Ron work through it at his own pace, he can usually find a way to make me understand. By the same token, if I push too hard, he becomes frustrated and that stress exacerbates the situation.

Ron also uses many gestures. It took some time to learn his gestures and their individual meanings, but we have developed an extensive vocabulary of gestures that we use regularly. You have to be with him and see him as well as his facial expressions to understand what he is trying to say, but it can be very effective. He tends to be very consistent, and some of his gestures are extremely humorous.

My career was going really well because I had recently found a new job at a company continuing my passion of implementation and training. However, just when we began to feel comfortable with our life and routine in Florida, an ominous but familiar cloud of loss began to hover over me with the death of my mother on January 5, 2006. This was an extremely painful time for me. My mother and I had a special relationship, and I could not imagine this world without her in it. Of all the losses I had experienced until then, I had never felt that level of anguish, knowing that I would never see my mom again. It seems that everyone experiences this kind of loss at one time or another, but I did not want to be a member of this universal group. I did not know how I would ever get over losing my mother or deal with the overwhelming grief that was drowning me, but having Ron in my life was comforting. He couldn't articulate the words that he wanted to say, but then, there are never appropriate words for this type of sadness. It just meant everything to be with him, feeling his solace with his embrace, and seeing the love he had for me in his eyes. We can never prepare ourselves completely for someone's death, but the month before, I wrote a special letter to my mother, expressing my love and appreciation for her, and I was able to read it to my mom prior to her death. Here are a few excerpts from that letter:

"You encouraged me to be a nurse and did not give up on me through all my years of education and jobs because you knew I was pursuing a dream. I'll never forget your face when I spoke about the art of nursing at my graduation from UNH. Aunt Blanche was a saint in your heart and I too wanted to be there. In any career, I will always be a nurse.

"You have taught me the important lessons in life: 'honor your father, be good to others, be honest, practice makes perfect, wash your hands, brush your teeth, and the most important—don't go to bed mad.'

"I am so grateful that you got to see my home in Florida, walk on the beach, and sit in my Jacuzzi to look at the stars. You knew this is where I was happiest. Although I moved many miles away, you knew my heart was always with you. I loved talking with you and Dad to let you know where I was at the time. You could always call that phone in my pocket and knew I was just a phone call away.

"You taught me to be honest in everything I do, whether it be with Ron, in my work, and even with you. The most difficult conversation I ever had was when we talked about your death. But you are ready and not afraid. You are facing death with such grace and honor. You said that it will be a relief to know that you are at peace as many others before you.

"My tears are tears of sadness knowing that I will no longer see you smile, hear your voice, or have you give me a reassuring touch. Just knowing that you have touched my life immeasurably, I will feel comforted by all the others that you have also touched.

"Thank you, I love you and I know God has blessed you."

Many never have the opportunity to say goodbye, and while it was not easy, I feel appreciative that I had that opportunity with my mother—rest in peace, Mom.

In 2007, we had lived in our home in Navarre for over two years. I continued to travel for work. We planned our summer vacations around our trips back to New Hampshire and Maine. We had sold our manufactured home, and we were renting a cottage in Maine for July and August that summer. This gave us plenty of time to visit with family and friends.

Earlier that year, during one of my numerous trips to Brooklyn, New York, Ron joined me. We had just arrived in our room, and as I was unpacking our bags, Ron fell to the floor and had a seizure. It only lasted for two minutes, but I panicked and called the front desk to request an ambulance. He was somewhat coherent. Several people came to the room wanting to see what happened. Ron managed his own medication, but we realized that in the excitement of making the trip, he forgot to take his medicine and thought that this was probably the cause of his seizure. Then the thought occurred to me that the tumor or cysts could have been coming back because he hadn't had surgery since 2000.

I needed to be at an agency the following day for work, but I had to let the boss know that I could not make it because Ron was with me, had a seizure, and I had to take him to the hospital. This ordeal was very scary. After a long stay in an overly congested emergency room in a Brooklyn hospital, they finally admitted Ron. This was his first seizure and I never felt so alone. I felt like Dorothy in the Wizard of Oz. I kept asking them to please call Boston. I hated the idea of Ron being in a strange hospital with an unfamiliar staff that did not have access to his medical records.

Their bedside manner wasn't that great, and he had more seizures while we were in the crowded ER. They asked me to leave him in this big room alone without anyone there with him, but I refused. Without knowing his medical history, coupled with his speech disability, they would never know what to do for him or what he needed. I understood his needs, I recognized his seizures, and I knew precisely what to do for my husband. There was no way on God's green earth that I was going to leave him alone in that horrible place.

It was probably eight hours before they finally found a bed for Ron, and he had three or four more seizures while we waited. I could not understand what was causing it, but knew he needed a dose of his seizure medication, which they reluctantly gave him after I made several requests. It was difficult to leave his side, not knowing what kind of treatment that he would receive. When the doctors there refused to call Boston and then suggested surgery, I called Boston. The doctor told me that they would just need the MRI results sent from Boston and they would do a comparison with their own assessment. Eventually they did their comparison and realized that Ron did not need a surgery. However, an increase in his medication was necessary.

In the days that followed, while he was in the hospital, I started a frantic price search to compare the cost of hotels and transportation to Boston. I felt like I was losing control, with seizures that could appear at any minute, risking injury to Ron if he fell. The writing was on the wall because this job was not going to work out for me anymore—not with Ron's condition as it was. New York was too far away, but if we could get a hotel in Boston, we would be close to Ron's doctor. However, not all of this was necessary.

It was hard to get people to understand our life and the daily dilemmas that bombarded our existence. Naturally, employers needed staff that they could rely upon, to go into work every day, at the same time, and stay until the scheduled ending time. As much as I wanted to make that commitment, as much as I needed to make that commitment, it was impossible because of the unpredictability that surrounded Ron's ever-changing condition.

Ron's seizures became more frequent. We tried the increased dosage of his seizure medication and monitored his response closely.

When we went to Maine for our vacation that year, Ron became weaker. While we were there, we took a trip down to Massachusetts, where we saw some friends who could also see that something was wrong. They confirmed my unspoken fear that it was time for yet another surgery. We made the appointment for his annual MRI, and they scheduled his surgery, which was successful. After Ron's recovery, we left the hospital and returned to the cottage in Maine. Home Health Services were available to help Ron with the weakness and function on his right side.

Upon our return to Florida, Ron continued his therapy as his dependence on me increased. Many wondered what I was going to do about work and the required travel because I needed to be available more for Ron. This meant a change in jobs, but I didn't know what would be available. I really liked my job with Allscripts, but I felt so overwhelmed. After many conversations with different managers, the company offered me a support position. This resulted in a pay cut, but I was able to work from home and be with Ron. Despite the change in pay, I've received several more benefits on a variety of levels, allowing me to utilize the many skills that I've gained throughout my career. My managers have been extremely supportive while helping me to find balance between life at work and at home.

The company mission statement continues to resonate within me—to be the most trusted provider of innovative solutions that empower all stakeholders across the healthcare continuum, to deliver world-class outcomes. I wonder how our lives could have benefited from all of Ron's care providers having access to the same medical records, MRI films, EEG tests, lab work, and medication lists. Allscripts is providing the ideal platform for a connected community, and I am proud to say that I am part of their organization. I cannot express how wonderful the manager was in helping me through the transition.

Unfortunately, earning less money quickly became a problem as Ron's medical bills were extensive, and I had exceeded my flexible spending account for that year. However, the bigger issue was managing the logistics of working from home. How could we live together and be in each other's space while I worked? It did not seem feasible, but I had to find a way to make it work—his safety and our finances depended upon it. I wondered how he felt about having to be so reliant upon me.

For as Long as we Both Shall Live

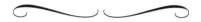

E very day has been a challenge to maintain my best "Wonder Woman" routine. I guess I live within a perpetual tug-of-war, trying to balance the needs of my husband with my own. Of course, it sounds like I'm painting a black and white picture of our life together, but there are so many other facets of our journey that make this the ultimate challenge, yet the most profound experience possible.

The average husband needs a wife who can share the nurturing, intimacy, and companionship that most couples naturally share. However, our situation is completely different from others because my husband needs so much more. What many take for granted is beyond precious to us. Our idea of romance is unconventional as Ron's physical limitations have altered our portrait of intimacy. Communication is a key element within any functioning relationship, but because of Ron's speech impairment, traditional dialogue between two people is not an option for us anymore. I would love to converse with my husband and best friend as we did before because throughout every challenge, every loss, and every beautiful element of life that we have shared together, we could talk to each other with trust and honesty without the worry of judgment from the other. Every fear or insecurity that I had developed as I grew into adulthood dissipated the moment I fell in love with Ron Gauvin. Sure, I had other fears and insecurities throughout life as anyone would, but he was truly the one who swept me off my feet and made me feel as though I was special, beautiful, and that anything in the world was possible.

I wish I could say that my emotions make sense, but considering the life we have had together, my emotions are anything but simple. I feel as though I have had to climb insurmountable mountains, yet the love I share with Ron was the reason I was able to climb those mountains. When I felt the worst frustration possible, even though it was with him at times, he was the one I have always wanted to confide in and talk out those frustrations. Again, his inability to communicate hindered that process, but with patience and a little creativity, we found a way to express ourselves to each other through gestures and alternative words from the norm. He clearly understands what I have to say, but because of the position of the tumor on his brain, reading and writing have become obsolete for Ron too. Clairvoyance or even mental telepathy would be extremely helpful in understanding all of the messages that Ron wants to share, but I managed to find my own extra sensory perception with him. I cannot say that I'm always right in interpreting what he wants to tell me, and I've realized that sometimes I need to exercise patience to give him the opportunity to demonstrate the thought he is trying to convey. However, overall, I understand him and I can hear his voice even in the most unconventional methods.

Now, I have a new set of fears because the love of my life believes in me, trusts me, and has the confidence that I can be and provide everything that he needs. This is a frightening prospect as I worry from day to day, as to whether I am making the right decisions for him or not. I have so much on my plate to do, to care for his daily necessities, to do my job effectively enabling me to pay our bills, and to find room for nurturing my own spirit and taking care of me. I constantly question myself wondering if I have the right to want "me" time or just a little escape from my daily reality. Is it wrong for me to need just a few moments to myself, to breathe in the ocean air and regroup for the next phase of life? Part of me feels as though it might be okay to want that for myself—that is, until something goes wrong.

I remember a time when Ron recently fell and hurt himself; it makes me nauseous just thinking of how serious it was and how serious it could have been. Ron took what we presumed to be a normal walk along his usual two-mile route. He was almost home, and then fell directly onto his face. Fortunately, a woman passing by found him, but he was lying in a pool of his own blood on the side of the road. Thank God, she thought to check his pockets and found his ID. Clearly, she knew what to do in a moment of crisis and did not panic. The first thing she did was call an ambulance, and then she came to our house and found me. I cannot even express the sheer terror that swallowed me when she came to the door and explained what had happened. I will be eternally grateful to her for her kind heart and altruism.

I wasn't sure what was worse—the fact that he fell, the uncertainty of his condition at that point, or that I was so busy in my own world working that I hadn't even realized that he was out on his walk. Of course, he took walks by himself before, but usually I had some awareness of his daily activities. This time, I became so involved in what I was doing, I forgot all about Ron.

As I rushed to the location where he fell, I could not help but feel an enormous amount of shame, guilt, and fear, because I wanted to have those moments to myself. I had to work to support us financially, but I felt selfish for wanting the little bit of escape that my work afforded me because clearly, it was to Ron's detriment.

I think I beat myself up more because Ron had fallen and bumped his head a week earlier while we were working out at the YMCA. Maybe I should have been even more aware after this recent fall, but it wasn't very serious. In fact, although the YMCA staff called an ambulance, it was apparent that he suffered only a minor bump and cut on his head, making it unnecessary for the ambulance to take him to the hospital. I had hoped that this fall would have been the same.

However, when I arrived to his location on the side of the road, I quickly realized that this was much more serious. The ambulance had arrived already and they had him strapped to a board wearing a neck brace. Blood covered his face and I could see a laceration over his left cheek, and another deep cut just under his nose, which was bloody and swollen. This was much more than I could have managed.

Because Ron had been having occasional seizures, I presumed that his fall resulted from another seizure. I explained Ron's history to the ambulance crew to help them while they treated him. Instead of riding in the ambulance, I drove to the hospital on my own because I wanted my car with me. The drive seemed like an eternity because I just wanted to be by his side. I hoped that he would not feel alone or remember any part of the ordeal.

When I arrived at the hospital emergency room, I refused to leave his side. The nurse in me felt compelled to help him and clean him up, but I knew I had to restrain myself and let the hospital staff do their jobs. It is amazing that we call it the (ER) emergency room when we have to wait for so long in most cases, but the wait was necessary because they ran an array of tests including X-ray, CAT scans, and extensive blood work. Fortunately, all of the results were negative and they let Ron come home.

When I think about that incident, I feel overwhelmingly sad for so many reasons. Ron needed time to recover from his fall and could not do the things that were part of his normal daily routine. He was in pain and needed medication to manage that pain. I felt the stress from everything I had to do, and at times, the walls seemed to be closing in on me. Then, I felt guilty for thinking of myself because he was so lost not being able to do the things he enjoyed doing.

I have to admit that some of our previous financial and weight struggles had stemmed from my desire to give Ron whatever he wanted. Both of us had suffered from increasing waistlines because we used to eat out a lot, and we chose foods that offered comfort over fitness. I've justified our lack of nutrition along with impulse purchases such as cars and vacations with the uncertainty of Ron's future. Not knowing how long he will be here, I just wanted to give Ron as much as possible and allow him to enjoy his life.

This has been such a lesson for me because despite everything, I've realized that if I don't take care of me, I cannot be any good to my husband. Consequently, I decided that I should go to the YMCA more often to work on my own health and fitness. It seems simple, but even working out at the "Y" presents challenges. If I go alone, I must worry about Ron being alone. If I take him with me, then I must focus my attention on his time there rather than my own.

One evening, I found myself sitting in the car, crying before driving home. Quite honestly, I just did not want to go home. I was there on my own, and I needed a little more time by myself before going back home. I have been going to the YMCA during the evenings just for a little while to get into better shape and to have a little time to myself. It has been therapeutic for me to get away without worrying that Ron would fall down, if he had been at the "Y" too. Whenever Ron was with me, I had to make sure he was exercising appropriately and I couldn't concentrate on my own routine. However, I still feel guilty for leaving him at home, by himself, while he patiently waits for dinner.

One day, I yelled at Ron and told him that I was tired of his moping around and feeling sorry for himself. Of course, I felt terrible immediately after, but my anger motivated Ron to do more. He started doing some of the household chores he had done previously, and he made an effort to be helpful to me as much as he could. I guess this was a positive result, but yelling at him did not make me feel as though I was helping him at all. I've always encouraged Ron's sense of independence by taking a rehab nurse approach to various aspects of his life. I thought it was important that he tried doing as much as he was capable of doing on his own, to prevent feelings of inadequacy or too much reliance upon me. However, I've always been more than willing to help if he asked for assistance with personal care or anything else that might require the use of two hands. Ron has become adept at tying his shoelaces with only his left hand, and although zippers are a bit of a struggle, if he persists, he usually gets it.

I have moments when I wonder what life would be like without Ron in my life and what I would do, but then, when I allow my mind to go to that place, it makes me feel terribly sad and I realize that I would miss him so much. I imagine how life would be in a variety of situations with Ron more dependent upon me and how I would handle it temporarily or indefinitely. However, I've learned that envisioning situations that do not exist is not productive or realistic, and I need to deal with our life as it is today, one day at a time. Making short-term plans makes more sense for us. I'm not afraid to look at the future with Ron, but I need to accept that I can only do the best I can with the circumstances that I have.

One of the primary issues that I needed to address was getting the doctors to consider prescribing Ron a different seizure medication or a higher dosage of his current one. His seizures had been creating risk for his well-being, cognitively, and physically because of his falling, which has happened more often than not. I knew that if I could get his seizures under control, Ron could function with more comfort and ease, and with less worry. I made an appointment with a local neurologist, and I requested his medical records from Boston to address this issue.

I feel as though I've grown quite a bit throughout our life together, especially after participating in a hospice volunteer training session, which was a requirement for hospice employees. The exercise was to recall my first experience with death, visualize death by thinking through what happens when someone dies, and discuss how I would like to die. In addition, the exercise asked what I thought I could do to make the thought of death less frightening, except this exercise was frightening as I looked at death in relation to Ron. I really didn't like this segment of the training, but I made an effort to get through it.

I was able to visualize Ron's final breath and then life without him. It sounds simple because it is not real, but when you allow your mind to go to that very dark place, it feels very real. The thought of life without Ron struck the most devastating emotions within me. I could feel the loss, the fear of being alone, and the question of what my life would mean without my husband. The pain I felt in that exercise made me realize that it would be significantly worse in real life. Still, I realized something else about myself while envisioning the worst scenario possible. I knew that Ron would not want my world to collapse. If I could not go on living my life after Ron's death, then everything I had experienced with him would have been in vain. The truth is that Ron taught me how to truly love and accept love. I have never given up on my husband, no matter how dire the circumstances seemed to be. What kind of person would I be if I gave up on myself after losing Ron? When I wasn't looking, he became my biggest life teacher, and I am who I am because of my life with Ron. After that exercise, I faced my worst fear, and I learned that despite the heartache I would feel losing Ron, it would not be nor should it be the end of my life.

Of course, Ron and I have had the morbid discussions that no one wants to have regarding end of life wishes. We talked about what he would want me to do if he was on life support without any chance of recovery or if he reached an irreversible state of delirium. Doctors always want to know if you want them to take extreme measures to resuscitate you if your heart stops. If not, they expect you to sign a Do Not Resuscitate (DNR) form, unless you prefer to leave the decision within the hands of your health care proxy or next-of-kin. These are terrifying circumstances to have to consider, but the doctors need to have a clear picture of your wishes to ensure they know precisely what to do in a moment of crisis.

Because of the serious nature of Ron's surgeries, we discussed these issues before every surgical procedure, knowing that there was always a risk involved. In addition, we talked about his preferred final arrangements after death. We had originally agreed that we both wanted cremation and to have our ashes scattered on an island in the West Indies. However, since we moved to Florida, we decided that we wanted some of our ashes thrown from the Navarre Beach Pier where we live, so we would always be together in spirit, in the paradise we found. Then, in honor of our parents, we also agreed that we wanted our remaining ashes buried at our family's burial plots, which happen to be in the same cemetery in New Hampshire.

After this death exercise, my previous fears have changed, and I am not afraid anymore. I realized that when you face death without fear, it liberates you to live life. I also learned that the idea of my husband's death did not have to be my focal point or daily dread. While I could imagine the horrible possibility, I needed to focus on today's reality, which is that my husband is here with me right now. He has exceeded expectations with his will to live. I could easily become one of those people who wore his death sentence upon their faces, but that is not who I want to be.

Another part of the hospice exercise was to reflect and share one of my earliest experiences with death. When I was only thirteen, my grandfather passed away. My parents would not allow me to visit the funeral home the first evening of calling hours. I have always maintained the thought that they were trying to protect me from seeing my dad cry. Oddly, I had never seen my father shed tears until my mother's funeral many years later. My father's inability to show his emotions while I was growing up made me want to marry a man who could share his sensitive side without fear. Because Ron's family displayed much of the same attitude as my family regarding their outward disapproval of men showing emotions, I thought it was important to encourage Ron to express himself and always share his feelings. He may not have had that same level of comfort with everyone, but during our quiet and private moments together, Ron has always trusted me enough to open his heart freely and express any emotion that he feels.

As a nurse, I have witnessed several patients who have died, and I was present for the death of my mom and Ron's dad. Arranging hospice services for each of them allowed me to be present until the end and care for their needs. It was an honor to be present during those sacred moments, and it helped to make those events real—seeing their final breaths of life. It was very comforting knowing that they were not suffering or alone. The one area that was difficult for me was the final zip of the body bag, and for some reason, I have never been able to watch the funeral home take away the bodies. However, I could handle and assist others through all of the other aspects of the death process.

I had three goals when I worked for hospice, which in retrospect, all met a need within me. First, I wanted to understand the financial aspects of hospice care. Then, I wanted to become proficient in handling pain management. Most importantly, I wanted to know that I was comfortable with the death of a patient. In reality, I wanted to know that I could handle the death of loved ones, if necessary. Reaching these goals has helped me immeasurably in work and in life, along with the side benefit of the volunteer training. While I enjoyed bedside nursing, I know that I would return to hospice nursing if the option was available to me.

I find myself reflecting upon many moments of my life with Ron especially during the past year. The year 2010 felt differently to me because I've been able to view all of Ron's experiences with eyes wide open and without the fear that used to plague me. Ron started having more falls, seizures, and even trouble holding his urine—the urgency he felt when he had to go to the bathroom was overwhelming and rapid. We had planned a road trip to New Hampshire and Maine for the summer, but considering the various issues he had been facing, the duration of a road trip that far away would not be feasible.

Improvising had become a way of life, so instead of letting that obstacle defeat us, we simply changed our road trip to flight plans. When arranging for a place to stay, I didn't want to reserve our usual blue cottage in Maine because I knew our stay would be tentative—contingent upon Ron's need for surgery. It was important that we take advantage of being near Boston if the opportunity to get Ron in surgery presented itself to us. A friend agreed to let us tentatively rent from her with a backup plan, if we had to be at the hospital for Ron's surgery. That kind of flexibility helped immensely. Then, with the plans for our trip north in place, I began to make arrangements for what I intuitively knew would be Ron's seventh surgery. Ron remembered previous surgeries, and he was afraid of the pain he might have to endure. I promised him that I would do everything I could to have the doctors give him plenty of amnesic drugs to prevent him from remembering the procedure or the pain. I knew how frightening this was for him, but the alternative to surgery was a wheelchair, to prevent Ron from getting hurt from possible falls, which was a scary prospect for both of us.

My objective was to go to Boston, suggest the surgery, and believe that this would solve all his problems. My way of thinking may have been a bit naïve, but I thought it was important to remain as positive as possible. Imagine my shock when I called Boston and discovered that Dr. Black was not at the practice anymore. This was a fear that had always sat in the back of my mind because doctors often change practices, or move to different hospitals and geographical locations. I had always hoped and prayed that Dr. Black would always be there for Ron. It took so much for me to trust the right doctor to operate on my husband's brain, and we had nineteen years of history with Dr. Black. Although Ron had experienced some right side paralysis after the initial biopsy surgery, amazingly, I never lost faith in Dr. Black or his ability to care for my husband. He was on the cutting edge of research and I wholeheartedly trusted him. I felt vulnerable not knowing anything about the new doctor, Dr. Johnson. To take some control over the helpless feeling I had, I began searching the internet for any information that I could find on this doctor. I learned that he has been practicing with Dr. Black since 2003. This made me feel a little better, but I planned to hold my judgment until I met him.

We scheduled the MRI for a Wednesday night at 6:30 p.m., which happened to be the same day as our flight into Boston. Of course, our plane landed at 5:00 p.m. that day, leaving very little margin for error. We immediately picked up a car, and I began driving to the hospital with barely a moment to breathe—at least that was my intention. It seemed the universe had other plans for us because I passed my exit at Prudential Center. It was an eastbound only exit and I was going west. It was already 6:20 p.m. and I was feeling a bit panicked. Fortunately, I saved the MRI receptionist telephone number, and I called to let her know where we were and that we would be there shortly. Sigh, I could see that it was not going to be that easy because my call went directly into voicemail. I left a message pleading for a return call, in hopes that someone would hear it and not cancel Ron's MRI.

Rush hour traffic in downtown Boston was insane, and I began to feel defeated, that is, until I saw a U-turn sign in the middle of the Mass Pike. That was a good sign, who knew! I immediately made the turn and I arrived at a crossroad of two choices. It had been a while, and I hoped that my memory would not let me down. I chose one of the Prudential Center exits and luckily, it brought me to Huntington Avenue. I knew my way from there—thank God!

Miraculously, we made it in time, and contrary to the earlier events of the day, the MRI was rather uneventful. Of course, it was easy for me to think that, considering I was not the one who had to receive a dye injection, and then lie motionless inside of a claustrophobic tube for forty-five minutes. Ron told me some time ago that during previous MRI tests, he was able to nap despite all of the loud noises. I suspect that after a day of flying in the air, and then in the car with me that he didn't have any difficulty falling asleep that time too.

Our friend Michele had offered her home in Boston as a respite, even though she had recently suffered major water damage and flooding in her basement. She was a generous soul, and she graciously gave us her bed for the night while she slept downstairs. She exemplified true friendship and helped me to realize that I could ask for help when I needed it. I don't think I truly understood how much I needed some girl friend time with Michele. Knowing we had a place to stay for the night relieved some of our stress, and having the opportunity to catch up with Michele and hear about some of her life's events was so refreshing. She had faced her fair share of challenges along the way, and it was intriguing to hear how she overcame those challenges. We discussed her recent weight loss and her quest to achieve a healthier lifestyle. I was excited about this because I had been working with Weight Watchers, trying to become more fit and healthy. Michele was amazing because she reached her weight loss goals and she became a runner in not just one, but three Boston Marathon races. It was so nice to chat with her about her life and not focus on our dilemma for a change. It was a welcomed distraction. Michele was so wonderful; she offered to have us back to stay at her place if Ron's doctor scheduled a surgery.

The next day, when we received the results of the MRI, the findings were not a surprise. I inquired about Dr. Black, but that information was not available to us. I mentally prepared myself for surgery, and I hoped that it would be better for Ron's quality of life. When we met Dr. Johnson, the new surgeon, he calmed my fears and agreed that Ron needed surgery. His nurse, Donna, whom we trusted had only good things to say about him. She had been with Dr. Black for as long as I could remember, and she really knew Ron.

I remembered thinking that if we could get the surgery done early, it would give Ron time to recover, and it would give us time to enjoy our vacation. When Dr. Johnson shared the results and his plan for surgery to remove cystic fluid from Ron's brain, he asked when we would like to do it. Without hesitation, I told him that Monday would be the best day for us. I had scheduled our flight home for the second day of August, which was eighteen days away. I wanted to have plenty of quality time together in Maine, and I selfishly wanted to celebrate my fiftieth birthday on the beach in Maine, eating a lobster roll.

With little time left before the unconfirmed surgery, we had several things to do. I had hoped that Dr. Johnson would approve having the surgery on Monday, and if that was an option, I needed to make sure the rest of our plans were in place. I spent the remainder of our trip back to New Hampshire reassuring Ron that we would get through this, and he just needed to be positive and have faith. My only regret was that I wish I had asked Dr. Johnson more questions about the surgery and Ron's concern about pain. Everything happened so quickly that I didn't follow my normal protocol.

Things were falling into place. We dropped off the rental car and boarded our scheduled bus heading north. Next was a call to my sister who was meeting us at the bus station in New Hampshire and letting us stay at her house for the night. Everything went smoothly, and we were on time for our meeting with her. Then, on Friday morning, we received the call that we were waiting for, telling us that they could schedule Ron's surgery for Monday, but they needed us back in Boston for the pre-op procedures. Of course, we left my sister's house in a whirlwind, and made it to Boston in excellent time.

When I try to recall those few days leading up to the surgery, it is still somewhat of a blur, but I managed to address everything on our list of things to do, including the arrangements for our accommodations before and after the surgery. Not to mention, we had to figure out what to do about my sister's vehicle and the parking in Boston. I think the worst part of the process was letting the rest of the family know we were back in New Hampshire for vacation, but also for Ron's surgery. I made many telephone calls and we shed a few tears.

Since I had been a regular blood donor, I arranged to donate blood during this pre-op visit. It really helped to know I was helping others, and it made me appreciate how fortunate we had been. There are so many who have depended upon a simple pint of blood, and I was happy to take a few minutes to do my part, which really put everything into perspective. I've always donated blood regardless of my own stress because I feel that this is an important gift. I also take time to donate platelets while Ron is having surgery. It helps pass the time and it is a great distraction.

Before returning to Boston for Ron's surgery, we moved from my sister's house to my friend's cottage in Maine. We stopped to have Ron's head shaved, which had become another one of our pre-surgery rituals. The hospital staff never seemed to do a very good job on his head, which caused Ron's hair to grow back uneven. Not to mention, they aren't always great at cleaning the blood from his scalp, but with a clean shave, I could take care of any other necessary grooming after his surgery.

We headed to the hospital on Sunday afternoon, and we chose to take a local commuter train from Maine to Boston, which would alleviate the worry of parking costs. When we arrived in Boston, we met our friend Michele first, and she took us out to dinner. She had invited us to come back and invade her home once again with open arms. It was such a nice feeling knowing we had an unconditional friend who never thought of our presence as an imposition. She opened her doors to us, and it gave us a little peace of mind. We spent much of the evening talking and mentally preparing Ron for his impending surgery.

Unlike Ron's previous surgeries, we found out that he did not have to be awake this time, which was a huge relief for him. It seemed that medical technology had advanced enough over the years to make it unnecessary to keep the patients awake for this type of procedure. Ron had been so afraid of the excruciating pain he would have to endure, yet again. I always felt helpless knowing what he was experiencing and not being able to do anything about it. That morning, he was able to smile with a huge sense of relief going into surgery because he knew that he could sleep through it and not feel any of the pain. While I waited during the surgery, I realized that I felt completely different from any other surgeries he had previously. I didn't have the same mounting fear that swallowed me in the past. I didn't feel the lump in my throat or the growing stomachache that never went away until he was in recovery. This time felt so different. I knew that he would come out of it just fine, and I knew that we had more time together. It was eerily calming to have that kind of awareness for the first time in almost twenty years, but I was right, Ron's surgery was successful with only minor problems. In Neuro-ICU, he was sleepy, but he was great! Dr. Johnson felt that the procedure went well and he was happy with the results. He drained the cyst, left the tube in, and added a reservoir for future draining. Ron's spirits were great and he felt so much relief that he slept through all of it and didn't feel any pain during the procedure. The only thing he remembered was counting backward—ten, nine, eight, seven—and lights out.

Amazingly, Ron had a voracious appetite and thirst already. This was an excellent sign. Unfortunately, two days later, he had a minor setback. We initially thought he was going to leave the hospital that day, but his brain was not ready. He tried to walk that morning, but he was unstable and shaky. In technical terms, his sodium level was off, and he needed to remain in the hospital until they felt satisfied that his levels were back to normal. Ron was in ICU, but it wasn't out of necessity. He was well enough to be in a regular room, but the hospital didn't have any available beds. Consequently, he had to stay in the private ICU room with the best nurses who welcomed my help in caring for Ron and assisting in communicating his needs.

The following day, Ron was amazing and back to his usual self, with only a minor headache. They discharged him that morning, and we spent the rest of our vacation time at the cottage in Maine while Ron recovered. It was a great way to celebrate my birthday, eating a lobster roll on the beach with a healthier Ron by my side. I felt such peace and serenity within, partly because of the ocean and partly because life felt completely different to me. I think Ron felt a new sense of inner peace this time too. Perhaps he came to it on his own, or it rubbed off me, but we were both feeling renewed, and it was invigorating.

We still face many challenges together and individually. While Ron's seizures seem to be in control now after changing his seizure medication he will always have certain physical limitations. It is difficult to imagine how all of this began nineteen years ago, when Ron received his initial diagnosis of a brain tumor and suffered from partial paralysis resulting from his biopsy. Those were the worst days of our married life together. It has certainly been a rough rollercoaster ride, but well worth it. We don't know what the future holds, but we have today—and today, despite everything that has occurred until now is a beautiful picture of love. To say that Ron is my beloved is an understatement because the fact is, he is the love of my life, and while I did not know my capacity for love, I found out throughout my journey with Ron.

I've learned so much about my husband, myself, and about healthcare. We grow up giving authority to many professionals in life, without fully realizing that these professionals are not perfect and they do make mistakes. It is so easy to accept a doctor's answer with his or her projected expiration date for the ones we love, without questioning it. Our society has always been willing to accept defeat and give up on the people whom we love when a healthcare professional makes a prognosis based upon straightforward clinical data—data that isn't always applicable to every case with different people and tenacity levels, varying body chemistry, and diverse environments.

I think that when we give up on the people we love, we are stealing their hope. Hope is what gives people the courage to fight for the things they want in life, and in this case, the courage to fight for life. Many doctors tell patients every day that they have a limited number of days, weeks, months, or years left to live—except many of those patients exceed those limitations and live for many more years. Who are we to take away the hope of someone who refuses to accept defeat? What gives doctors the right to disregard a patient's will to live?

I cannot express the number of times I've seen tragic expressions on the faces of a new rotating residents, interns, or nurses, when they discovered that Ron had a brain tumor. It was as if they immediately dismissed any chances of recovery or extended life because of his condition, without taking the time to familiarize themselves with him or his complete medical history. It was bad enough that I had seen their negative expressions, but it wasn't fair that Ron had to see death prematurely staring back at him through their unaware eyes. The sad part was that they didn't have the slightest clue of how he had beat every odd, exceeded every expectation, and lived because he wanted to live. Ron is the very reason why healthcare professionals publish their astounding discoveries and extraordinary feats in medical journals.

As a nurse, I understand that doctors must remain detached to a certain degree, and I understand that their part in all of this is on a clinical level, but sometimes they are downright cold and indifferent, with little sensitivity or compassion for the one, who they just stamped with an expiration date.

"I don't want to give false hope, or you are in denial." How many times have I heard that? I don't believe there is any such thing as false hope. Those combined two words represent an oxymoron, in my humble opinion. There isn't anything false about hope, as it represents truth in its purest form. Hope is a fusion of trust and faith in the seemingly impossible—it is what a patient or individual must have to move forward in this life. If sick people didn't have a reason to hope, they wouldn't fight to live. Doctors feel stymied by the miracle of life when it is not consistent with their scientific statistics or clinical evidence. The funny thing is that you cannot learn that aspect of healing in medical school because those are the lessons that you learn through life's formidable experiences.

I learned many lessons regarding loss and grief, and I learned something even more about the value of life just by living with and caring for my husband. There were times when I questioned Ron's positive outlook, along with his other coping methods, but my husband's courage and positive outlook enabled him to continue living. Even though some doctors have told me I was in denial, Ron has been living proof that with unwavering determination, anything is possible. We struggled, we communicated, we stopped communicating, and then, we reinvented ways to communicate again. Through every word and every silence, we remained true to our vows and united as an unbreakable promise.

The hardest part of loving someone is having the courage to let them love you back, but Ron gave me that courage, and through a mountain of challenges and losses, we have prevailed because the blissful moments in our life have given us hope through the eyes of our love.

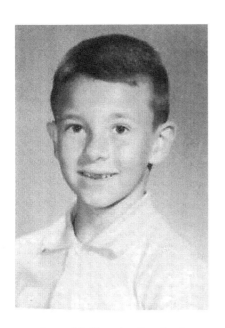 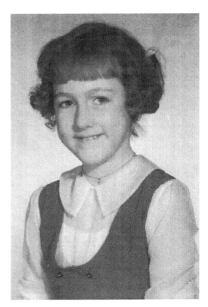

Ronald Gauvin Grade 2   Patricia Meserve Grade 2

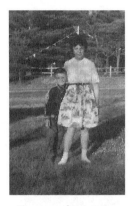

Ron and Joanne

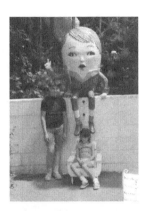

Story Land, NH
Ron and Dianne

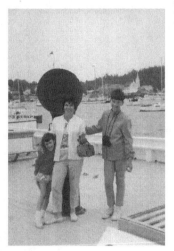

Booth Bay Harbor, ME
Dianne, Mom, Ron

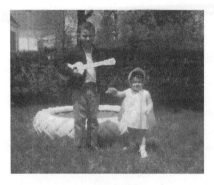

Ron and Dianne

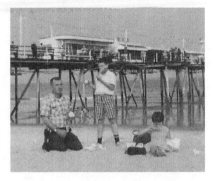

Old Orchard Beach, ME
Dad, Ron, Dianne

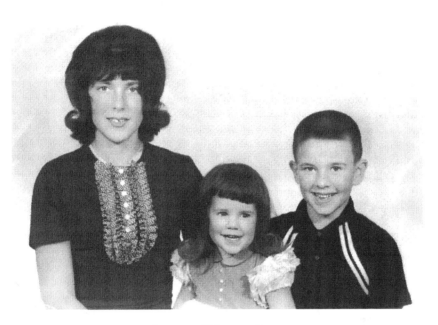

Joanne, Dianne, Ron

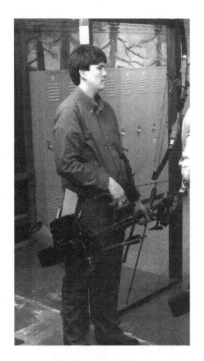

Archery Tournament

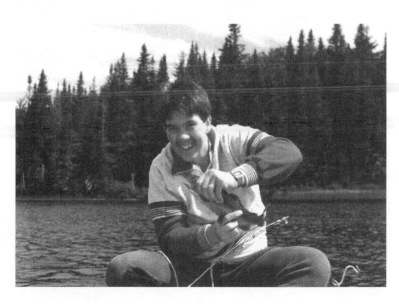

Fishing with Dad

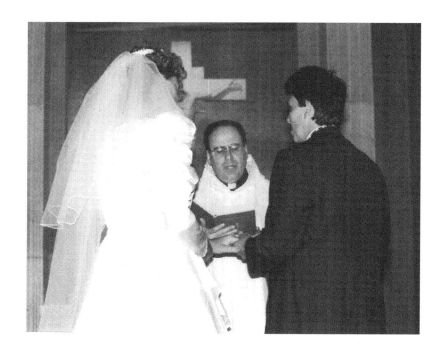

Wedding Vows

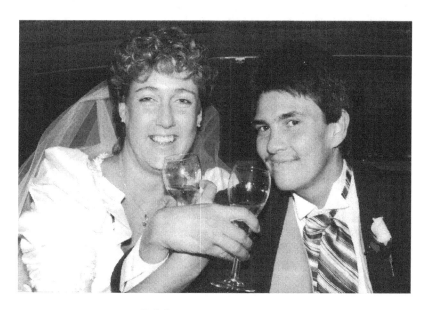

Celebrating our Marriage

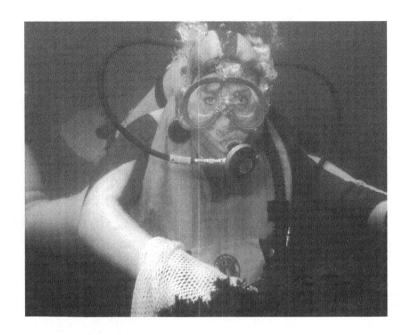

Patti scuba diving

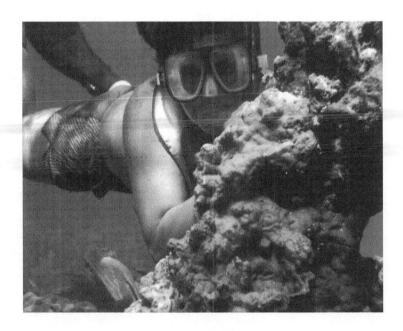

Ron snorkeling

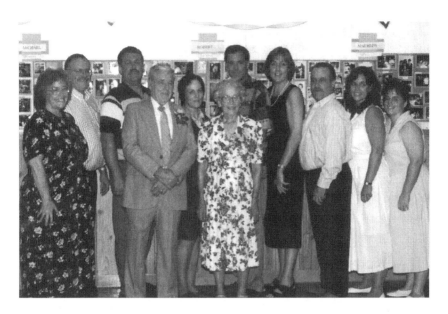

Patti's Family

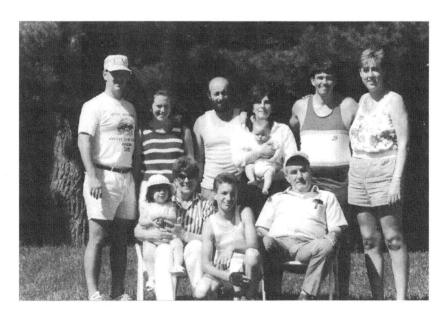

Ron's Family

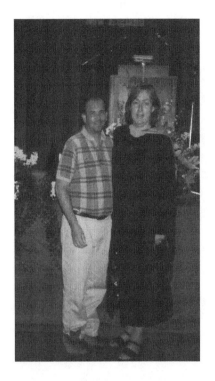

Ron and Patti Graduation
Antioch

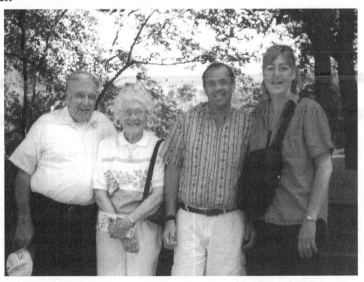

Mom & Dad Meserve, Ron and Patti in NYC

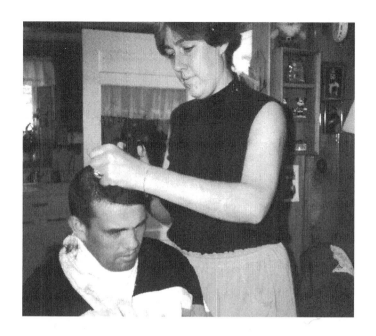

Shave prior to surgery, 1994

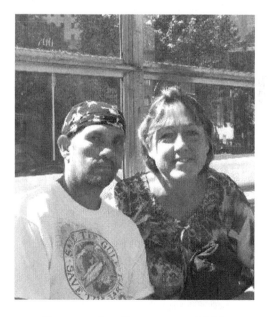

Boston trip after surgery 2010

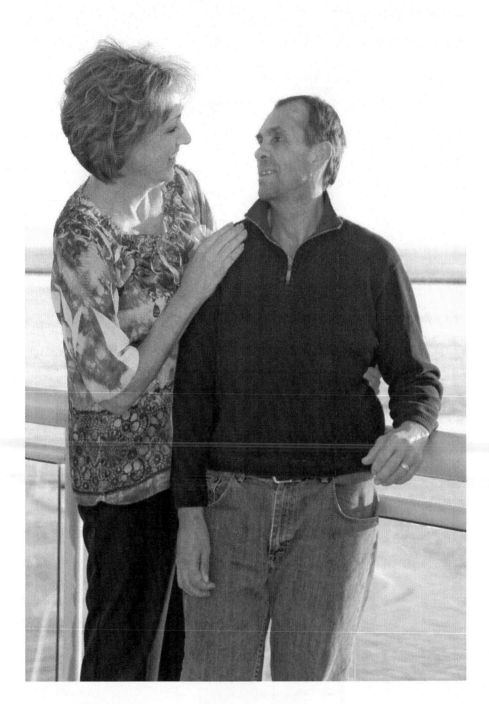

Ron & Patti